Cultural Competence in Health Care

Wen-Shing Tseng • Jon Streltzer

Cultural Competence
in Health Care

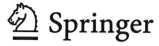 Springer

Wen-Shing Tseng, M.D.
University of Hawaii School of Medicine
Honolulu, Hawaii
TsengW@dop.hawaii.edu

Jon Streltzer, M.D.
University of Hawaii School of Medicine
Honolulu, Hawaii
streltzerj@dop.hawaii.edu

ISBN 978-0-387-72170-5   e-ISBN 978-0-387-72171-2
DOI: 10.1007/978-0-387-72171-2

Library of Congress Control Number: 2007943038

Preface

Modern medicine is making remarkable advances associated with breakthroughs in medical technology and rapidly accumulating biomedical knowledge. However, it is a commonly shared concern that, in becoming more technically oriented, the practice of medicine—with a sometimes excessive focus on the body while ignoring mind and emotion—struggles to maintain a human face. There is a strong need to correct this skewed tendency and to practice medicine that emphasizes the integration of mind and body—to see and care for the patient as a whole person— a spirit endorsed by the contemporary field of psychosomatic medicine. As an extension of this, there is an urgent need to provide culturally competent care for patients—that is, care that is concerned about cultural issues—and tailors interactions and interventions in ways that appropriately takes culture into account. Societies around the world, including ours, are becoming multiethnic and polycultural. The reality of medical care is that we treat people of diverse backgrounds with varying customs and beliefs.

Inequalities of care among minorities and the culturally different are being increasingly documented. As a result, the Surgeon General of The United States has recently urged that medical care become increasingly culturally competent. A major goal in solving this problem is the inclusion of a cultural focus in medical education. A rapidly increasing number of training programs are requiring that cultural competence training be included in their curricula. Despite this, books addressing this topic are few. This book, *Culture Competence in Health Care: A Guide for Professionals*, is intended to fill this void for students of medicine, nursing, social work, clinical psychology, and other healthcare disciplines. It is designed to be helpful for practicing physicians and health practitioners, in general. Objectives of this book include providing critical knowledge about cultural issues in healthcare, approaches to obtaining necessary cultural knowledge in specific situations, and enhancing cultural sensitivity by stressing the cultural implications of various interactions and situations in healthcare settings.

This book is written as a joint collaboration of two authors—one (Tseng) specializes in cultural psychiatry and the other (Streltzer) specializes in consultation-liaison psychiatry. By combining our experience and expertise in these two areas, we have developed and organized a new body of knowledge into this book addressing the issue of the cultural aspects of healthcare. We have worked together to publish several books in the past, including: *Culture and Psychopathology* (Bruner/Mazel, 1997), *Culture and Psychotherapy* (American Psychiatric Press, 2001), and *Cultural Competence in Clinical Psychiatry* (American Psychiatric Publishing Inc., 2004). This book is a continuation of our collaboration—a further stage in our work on culture and clinical care.

The book consists of nine chapters, covering culture and healthcare from several perspectives. It provides an overview of the concept of culture, and it discusses key issues in various medical and healthcare specialties. The book reveals the way culture influences interactions with patients, including how to use interpreters to overcome language barriers. A chapter is devoted to cultural issues in working with patients of selected ethnicities. The book covers special medical issues and certain medical diseases. Cultural influences on mental disorders are reviewed. The final chapter summarizes the main themes addressed in the book with specific suggestions for providing culturally competent health care for patients in general.

We have attempted to strike a balance in the subject matter between clinical application and theoretical elaboration. In many chapters, case vignettes are inserted to illustrate the issues elaborated in the text. Most of them are based on actual cases encountered by the authors or contributed by colleagues. Appropriate modifications have been made in the consideration of confidentiality. The material of the book has been derived primarily, but not entirely, from research and experiences in the United States, but the basic principles will apply to medical practice in a variety of cultural settings that are applicable to healthcare professionals around the world as well.

Wen-Shing Tseng, M.D.
Jon Streltzer, M. D.

Contents

Chapter 1
Culture and Medical Practice

What Is Culture?

Healthcare providers must understand what culture is to perform culturally competent medical care for patients of diverse ethnic, cultural, or minority groups. Several related terms such as race, ethnicity, minority, and social class must be recognized and distinguished. Let us first define what culture is.

Culture

Culture refers to the unique behavioral patterns and lifestyles shared by a group of people that distinguishes that group from others. Culture is characterized by a set of views, beliefs, values, and attitudes toward life that is transmitted from generation to generation. Culture may be expressed in various ways that regulate life—through customs, etiquette, taboos, or rituals. It is manifested in the activities of daily life and reflected in cultural products, such as common sayings, legends, drama, art, philosophical thought, religions, and political and legal systems. Culture influences health and illness in the ways people conceptualize a given illness, seek help, utilize the healthcare system, relate to healthcare providers, and accept medical treatment prescriptions.

In practice, the identification of the cultural background of an individual can be problematic, because the impact of culture can be conscious or unconscious (in other words, the person may or may not be aware of it). Culture is abstract and can be amorphous; is not static over time and is often in flux (that is, subject to cultural change over time and through different generations); and its impact on subgroups of people (even those living within the same society) may vary greatly within subcultures.

Language is one of the instruments through which culture is transmitted and expressed. Through language, a person communicates not only semantic meanings, but also underlying conceptions, values, and attitudes that can be very different among different cultural systems. Comprehending another person's culture through his or her language can therefore be quite challenging, particularly when that language is very different from one's own.

W.-S. Tseng and J.M. Streltzer (eds.), *Cultural Competence in Health Care*
© Springer 2008

Race

The term *race* is quite different from culture. In the past, race has been used to refer to a group of people that is characterized by certain common physical features, such as color of skin, eyes, and hair, facial or body features, or physical size. On the basis of these physical features, one group is distinguished from other groups. It was once considered that race was attributed to biological factors. In the past, anthropologists have used the term *geographic race* to indicate a human population that has inhabited a continental landmass or an island chain sufficiently long to have developed its own distinctive genetic composition compared with that of other geographic populations (Hoebel 1972). However, recent advances in genetic studies analyzing DNA among members of different races have shown that there are greater variations within racial groups than *between* them (American Anthropological Association, 1999). Thus, it is now thought that races are socially and culturally constructed categories that may have little to do with actual biological differences. From a medical point of view, race is continuously used to differentiate groups of people who may have different susceptibilities to certain kinds of medical diseases. For example, people of African descent tend to suffer more from sickle cell anemia and people of Asian background are plagued more by pharyngeal or stomach cancer.

Ethnicity

Ethnicity refers to social groups that distinguish themselves from other groups by a common historical path, behavioral norms, and their own group identities. Members of an ethnic group are affiliated and may share a common language, religion, culture, racial background, or other characteristics that make them *identifiable* within their own group. Thus, culture refers to manifested characteristic behavioral patterns and value systems, while ethnicity refers to a group of people that share a common cultural feature or root culture. Because culture is abstract—difficult to recognize and identify—ethnicity is used instead for identification. However, ethnicity is not exactly the same as culture. An ethnic group may have different subcultures, while different ethnic groups may share a common culture.

Minority

A minority is a relatively smaller group that is identified in relation to a majority group in society. Strictly speaking, minority groups may not automatically suffer from social disadvantages. In fact, some minorities have more privileges and enjoy more social achievements than the majority. However, in most cases, minorities encounter mistreatment by the majority and suffer from discrimination and social disadvantage. Thus, minority peoples often hold resentment toward the majority, whether openly expressed or unspoken. The concept of a *minority* is a social one, often related to economic or occupational factors that may or may not be related to matters of ethnicity or culture. Many people with physical handicaps (such as deafness, mute or blindness), or with socially stigmatized medical diseases (such as leprosy or AIDs) may be discriminated against by others and suffer from being a minority with social disadvantages.

Social Class

This refers to the subgroups that exist within a given society, usually due to different economic or occupational factors. People of different social classes may live in different areas geographically, maintain different styles of social interaction, and enjoy different social facilities. Ethnic or racial background may be additional factors that contribute to such social segregation or differentiation. People from a given social class may have their own subculture that is different from other social classes, and they may or may not be aware of the existence of such differences. In America, with our egalitarian ideals, we tend to deny the existence of social class in our society, even though in reality subtle or obvious social class differences exist at any given time. In regard to health and sickness, it is the general pattern that underprivileged classes tend to have less opportunity to access proper healthcare and, as a result, suffer more from medical problems.

Culture and Illness Behavior

Illness behavior refers to how patients think, react, and cope when they suffer from illness. It includes how they perceive and understand their sickness, seek help for their health problems, utilize healthcare systems, and how they benefit from healthcare. In contrast to this, *health behavior* refers to how people behave to maintain their health. This may include how people follow guidance on food intake, exercise, hygiene, preventive exams, and so on. A patient's illness or health behaviors are subject to individual factors such as education and past experiences, as well as cultural factors, and these elements may need to be recognized to properly understand the patient.

How physical dysfunctions are perceived and managed differently by various ethnic groups is shown in the study carried out by Zuckerman, Guerra, Drossman, Foland, and Gregory (1996). They conducted a survey of a nonpatient population in Texas to examine ethnic differences of healthcare-seeking behaviors related to bowel dysfunction. They reported that Hispanic-Americans, who tend to see bowel dysfunction as a daily issue, were less likely to seek healthcare for such. Furthermore, they were more likely to self-medicate with folk remedies to maintain good bowel function. In contrast, nonHispanic (Caucasian) Americans tend to see bowel dysfunction as a medical problem requiring a visit to a physician for a prescription.

The Distinction between "Disease" and "Illness"

Although the terms *disease* and *illness* are semantically synonymous, cultural anthropologists and cultural psychiatrists make an important distinction between them. *Disease* is taken to refer to the medical definition of sickness by professionals, and is explained from the perspective of biological and physiological etiology, patterned clinical manifestations, course, and outcome. Disease is considered objective and universally similar in nature. In contrast, *illness* refers to the patient's psychological construct of the perception, experience, and understanding of suffering. Illness is subjective and open to cultural impact.

For instance, a man suffers from epileptic seizures. A physician conceptualizes it as a medical *disease* occurring as a result of focal electrical discharges in the brain causing central nervous system dysfunction. Medication is needed to control such a disease, otherwise it will recur and may cause serious injury to the patient. From the patient's point of view, the seizure is an *illness* that may occur suddenly, and may or may not interfere with daily behavior. It might be interpreted as a minor annoyance, or it might be interpreted as the result of a force imbalance in his body—a temporary possession by an evil spirit, or the consequence of an ancestor's immoral behavior. The illness is a disgraceful condition that needs to be hidden from others, otherwise it may affect the patient's future life in areas such as work or marriage.

The example of the epileptic patient illustrates that the *disease* is the concept utilized by modern medical personnel, while the *illness* is the concept used by the common people. These two concepts may or may not overlap in some ways, but in many ways they are different. From a cultural point of view, a physician needs to know and comprehend the whole situation—not just the medically oriented concept of the disease, but also the patient's and his family's perception of the illness.

Folk Concepts and Explanations of Illness

People usually have common knowledge of—and hold certain beliefs about—illness. These can be *folk* or *old housewife* cures based on accumulated past experience or well-established traditional medical concepts that have deep roots in the society. Based on the nature of the explanation, these can be discussed from supernatural, natural, or somato-medical perspectives.

Supernatural Explanations

These explanations are based on supernatural beliefs. They attribute the causes of sickness to supernatural powers that are beyond human understanding and control. Explanations such as these are often utilized when the occurrence of sickness is beyond an ordinary person's understanding. Supernatural explanations of illnesses take many forms.

Object Intrusion

In a concrete way, sickness is interpreted as the result of the intrusion of certain undesirable objects, such as tiny bones, bits of leather, coagulated blood, insects, or hairs. All are considered evil and are proven to be the causes of illnesses in concrete and convincing ways by people who believe in this theory. It is based on magical thought, which is different from the nature-orientated pathogenic object theory. According to Clements (1932), this is perhaps one of the most primitive ways of interpreting the causes of sickness.

Soul Loss

Soul here refers to the supernatural being of *self*, which usually resides in our bodies. This is a view held by many people in preliterate societies. It is believed that for some reason, such as being frightened, hit on the head (where the soul resides), sneezing, or experiencing troubled sleep, the soul leaves the body and is unable to return. It is thought that when a person has lost his individual soul, he will become sick.

Spirit Intrusion

This explanation takes the view that sickness is due to the presence in the body of evil spirits. Although the presence of spirits or other supernatural beings does not necessarily cause sickness all the time, the intrusion of malicious spirits does.

Breach of Taboo

This explanation sees sickness as a punishment by the gods for the breach of religious prohibitions or social taboos that have divine sanction. The breach may be unintentional or even unknown to the sufferer, but is still interpreted as the cause of the illness. Voodoo death is often attributed to *breach of taboo*. According to this interpretation, there are certain ways to undo the punishment, including confession.

Sorcery

This interpretation considers sickness to be the result of the manipulations by persons skilled in magic or having supernatural powers. It is suspected that illness is induced with malicious intent by the acts of others, through the use of supernatural powers. Repairing troubled interpersonal relations is one way to remove the effects of the sorcery—performing counteracting sorcery is another.

Natural Explanations

These explanations stem from the basic assumption that there are underlying principles of the universe that govern all of nature—including health and sickness. When physical illness occurs, the causes are thought to be related to natural matters in several ways.

Disharmony of Natural Elements

It is assumed that certain homeostatic conditions exist in the world of nature by means of the harmonic balancing of various elements. If there is disharmony among these natural elements, illness as an undesirable condition will occur. The humoral view of Greek medicine and the five-element theory of Chinese medicine are both rooted in this basic concept.

Incompatibility with Natural Principles

Closely related to the concept of the correspondence between microcosm and macrocosm, some people believe that illness is brought about by incompatibility with natural principles. Astrologers may interpret sickness as the result of unusual movement by one's designated star in the sky. Geometrists (or *feng-shui* masters) may explain that you suffer from a chronic illness because your ancestor was buried in a place that does not fit geometric, or *feng-shui*, principles. A fortune-teller may interpret that one has excessive fire or water in the body system, or that one's yin and yang are not properly balanced.

Noxious Factors in the Environment

In this view, when any natural element, such as wind or water, is excessive or unnatural, it becomes noxious and causes illness. Cold air is considered to be the cause of *catching cold*, even in contemporary times. Apoplexy was thought to occur as the result of the intrusion of *wind* in Chinese medicine. Thus, the condition was labeled *zhong-fun*, which literally means *attack by wind*.

Somato-Medical Explanations

This group of explanations views sickness as the result of undesirable conditions existing within our own bodies. It considers certain conditions necessary for the organism to function. Any factors that are not favorable to these conditions will result in sickness.

Distress or Dysfunction of Certain Visceral Organs

This explanation is based on the belief that certain visceral organs are closely related to certain physical and mental functions. Due to distress or other reasons, dysfunction of particular organs may occur, which in turn leads to certain somato-emotional disturbances. The heart distress conceived by Iranian people (Good 1977), the kidney-deficiency syndrome of the Chinese (Wen 1995), and neurasthenia (exhaustion of the nervous system) diagnosed by physicians and believed by people in the West at the turn of the 19th century, are some examples.

Physiological Imbalance or Exhaustion

A badly balanced diet, exhaustion, or inappropriate activity, especially sexual, is considered to cause physiological disturbances that result in medical disorders. Loss of energy through excessive sexual activity has been held responsible for unhealthy conditions in both the Eastern and the Western worlds. An elevated fire element in the body (labeled *hwa-byung* by Koreans), causing irritability and anger as well as other somatic dysfunction, is another example.

Based on the Greek humoral concept of pathology, according to which the four bodily fluids or *humors* were characterized by a combination of hot or cold with wetness or dryness, people in Latin America today classify most foods, beverages, herbs, and medicines as *hot* or *cold*. By extension, illness is often attributed to an imbalance between heat and cold in the body (Currier 1966).

Insufficient Vitality

It is believed that a person, as an organism, needs a certain force, vitality, or energy to function. Many terms have been used to describe the concept of such a force or vitality in different societies, such as *mana* for Hawaiians, *Jing* and *qi* for Chinese, *dhat* for Indians, *genki* for Japanese, and so on. No matter what term is used, the basic underlying concept is that it is important to acquire, maintain, and reserve this biological-mental force for a person to function effectively. If there is insufficiency or excessive loss of the force, it will often result in sickness, and a resupply of the force will be needed.

Traditional Medicine: Theory and Practice

Traditional medicine refers to the medical system that has been developed, existed, and was practiced in the past prior to the development of *modern medicine*. The concept and theory of sickness and treatment for it may differ considerably from that of modern medicine. However, many people in our society still strongly believe in and practice traditional medicine—either separately or concomitantly with modern medicine.

Traditional Chinese medicine practiced in China (as well as other parts of Eastern Asia, such as Japan or Korea), Ayurvedic medicine practiced in India, and Galenic-Islamic medicine observed by the Arabian people, are some of the traditional medical systems that are well-elaborated with theory. Such beliefs are deeply held by many patients and families. Therefore, it is important for the modern healthcare professional to have some basic knowledge about traditional medicine so that appropriate care can be formulated and delivered to such patients.

For example, patients of Asian backgrounds may automatically accept the yin and yang theory of traditional Chinese medicine. Patients may inquire whether it is all right to eat certain fruits after childbirth or surgery because this relates to the yin and yang theory. Some families may scratch a child's body with a coin to create a *fire-elevated* condition. Physicians not familiar with this folk treatment may wrongly interpret ecchymotic skin injuries as a sign of child abuse. Burn scars on the back or the belly of a patient may puzzle the physician if he or she does not recognize this as the result of *oqiu* treatment (moxibustion), which some cultures use to treat stomach disorders, back pain, or cancer.

Culture of Patients, Physicians, and "Medical Culture"

In a medical setting, three types of culture are present and interact with each other—namely, the culture of the patient, the culture of the physician, and a specific medical culture.

The Culture of Patient

The culture of the patient contributes to the patient's understanding of an illness—the perception and presentation of symptoms and problems—and the adjustment to the illness. The patient's expectations of the physician, motivation for treatment, and compliance are also influenced by the culture of the patient.

The Culture of Physician

This refers to the cultural system held by the physician (or other healthcare professionals). It superimposes itself on the physician's personality traits, personal beliefs, and professional knowledge, and will shape the pattern of interaction and communication with the patient. For example, a physician may be influenced by cultural prejudices or biases toward a particular gender (male/female differences), sexual orientation (gay/lesbian), race or ethnicity, specific disease (AIDs/alcohol abuse), or certain medical procedures (abortion/euthanasia).

The Medical Culture

This refers to traditions and practices that have developed within the medical service setting beyond medical knowledge and theory. Whether the physician and nurse work together as egalitarian team members or in a strictly hierarchical order depends on the medical culture, as does society's choice of a socialized or privatized medical system. On a clinical level, a patient can be informed about a fatal illness or the actual diagnosis can be concealed from him with the idea of protecting a *vulnerable* patient.

Examining medical practice in America, anthropologist Stein (1993) observed that being in control is very important for the American doctor. The physician's dominant values are individualism (the doctor can do it himself), mastery over nature (he can cure the disease), and future orientation (focused on the patient's eventual cure). Active intervention, aggressive treatment, control, and fixing the patient above all else are accepted attitudes and morale for the clinician—strongly reflecting American value systems that may not necessarily be shared in other cultures.

To provide culturally appropriate care, it is essential to recognize how cultural factors may influence the patient, physician, medical staff, and medical setting. Based on such knowledge, we can then proceed to the practical aspects of treatment.

The Relationship Between Medical Providers and the Patient

The Physician-Patient Relationship

In response to an acute illness, the physician and patient establish a relationship in which the physician-healer functions in an authoritative role, taking responsibility for the treatment plan. The patient, in the role of the one being healed, takes a position of dependence on the physician and is a passive participant in the healing process. This is exemplified by an extreme situation, such as a major operation performed under general anesthesia. Once the patient agrees to accept such a healing procedure, he becomes entirely passive under general anesthesia. The surgeon takes an active role in performing the surgical procedure, thus becoming responsible for all activity regarding the patient.

Beyond this basic physician-patient relationship, the healer-client relationship is subject to cultural variations—particularly if the illness is more chronic, where the healer does not rapidly provide a cure. For example, the extent to which the physician can act in an authoritative role rather than a more egalitarian one is influenced by the cultural system and how authority is assigned to the healing profession.

The general tendency is that if a society is autocratic and the leaders—such as the head villager, police, or governmental administrator—are authoritative, then the physician can also exercise more power in relating to the patient. In contrast, if the society is democratic, the physician tends to show more respect for the rights of the patient and relates to the patient in a more egalitarian way.

Patient's Relation with the Medical Team

In the medical system, there are personnel with various levels of training, including doctors, nurses, medical technicians, bedside nursing aides, and social workers. Members of the medical team relate to each other, and the team hierarchy is maintained in a manner based not only on treatment needs but also on a medical culture that, at least in part, reflects the general culture in the society. In Japan, for example, physicians are typically male and the nurses are female. The nurses are expected to bow to the physicians and to treat them as masters, thus reflecting the traditional hierarchy in Japanese society where men occupy a superior position to women. In contrast, although American nurses are required to carry out the physicians' medical orders, they are usually given a certain amount of power in carrying out their functions. As the major figures in charge of the wards, nurses can make suggestions to physicians—sometimes strongly—on the management of patient care. Consciously or subconsciously, physicians have to relate to nurses in the same way that men are supposed to relate to women in American society—with respect and on an equal basis.

Dealing with medical teams with different power structures, patients will learn and adjust to each team. For example, Japanese patients will hesitate to ask questions or make requests directly to the authoritative physician and instead will try to go through the nurses, with whom they feel more comfortable sharing any problems. In contrast, American patients do not feel the need for such an indirect approach. They will usually communicate directly with the physician concerning their diagnosis or treatment plan, and with nurses on other issues such as what medication the doctor has prescribed. They recognize the different roles performed by various members of the medical team and will interact with them accordingly. However, if a Japanese patient were to be hospitalized in an American hospital, he or she may be confused as to how to relate appropriately to the medical team and come across as a passive, stoic, or uncomplaining patient. If an American patient was admitted to a Japanese hospital, the patient—without knowing it—may behave in a way that would be interpreted as too direct and aggressive in relating to the physician.

Not all societies have primarily male physicians and female nurses. In Russia, the majority of physicians are women, and in the United States, many men work as nurses. The gender distribution of physicians has also changed with time. An example is the United States, where obstetricians and gynecologists were predominately male doctors a generation or two ago, but are now primarily female. How the gender of the physician and nurse influences the medical situation is a challenging question. For instance, how female physicians relate to female nurses or how male physicians relate to male nurses is part of a distinct medical culture, albeit influenced by the dominant societal culture.

Patient's Commitment to a Physician

In the United States and many other Western societies, the medical systems and cultural values expect that a person has an established family physician who sees them for care. If there is a need for a specialist for a second opinion, the family physician will usually recommend one, and the patient usually follows the recommendation. The general rule is that the patient sticks to one family physician with a commitment to a long-term relationship and seldom changes physicians unless there is a specific reason for doing so.

In other societies, such as many Asian countries, a patient will shop around for physicians without feeling a commitment to remain with any particular family physician. The patient may rely on a friend or relative's recommendation to see a particular physician—usually one with a good reputation in the patient's or family's point of view. However, there is no long-term commitment, and very often a patient may see several physicians simultaneously or change to another physician. It is not uncommon for a patient to see modern and traditional physicians at the same time. Therefore, a modern physician would not get too upset upon finding out that the patient is concurrently seeing another physician. It is mainly a matter of the patient's concept of commitment and does not reflect on the patient's respect of the physician.

Patient's Satisfaction with Physician

A patient's satisfaction with the physician is determined by many factors, including how the physician relates to the patient, to what extent explanations are given, and the kind of support given to the patient. Therefore, a patient's satisfaction with the physician may not correlate with the actual success of the medical treatment.

In Israel, Baider, Ever-Hadani, and De Nour (1995) carried out a cross-ethnic comparative study of cancer patients' satisfaction with their physicians. The study compared Israeli veterans and Russian patients who had immigrated to Israel within the past four years. Patients were asked to describe the *actual* physicians they had encountered and their *ideal* physician with the index for satisfaction based on the similarities between the two descriptions. The Russian patients had significantly higher satisfaction scores compared to their Israeli counterparts. There was no reason to suspect that the Russian patients had greater success with their medical treatments than the Israelis, therefore how the patients' satisfaction was affected by their ethnic backgrounds, past medical experiences, or current medical expectations, deserves further study.

Privacy and Confidentiality

Between patient and physicians there is the matter of how to provide privacy in examining the patient and keep things confidential regarding any information obtained from the patient. These medical-ethical matters are subjected to cultural influences and modification.

Privacy

It is almost an unspoken rule in contemporary (Western) hospitals that privacy needs to be considered and observed. For example, when an obstetric-gynecological doctor performs an examination of a (female) patient, it needs to be performed in an examination room with privacy. If the doctor is male, a female nurse is usually present in the room. However, for Muslim married female patients, the husband expects to be present in the room when the examination is performed. For Micronesian unmarried female patients, it is necessary to invite their mothers or sisters to be present in the room. Therefore, the degree of privacy is different according to the specific culture.

Confidentiality

To what extent medical issues are kept confidential with the patient or his family, as well as to outsiders is a sensitive issue which varies from culture to culture. For American culture, which emphasizes individuality, a pediatrician no longer automatically shares medical information with parents when a youth reaches the age of 16, and may confine important information to the patient only. However, for many conservative societies in which the concept of family is greatly emphasized—and parental authority is greatly valued—parents expect to know everything about their children no matter how old their children are. If a doctor shares the findings only with the patients, and does not share with the parents, the parents will feel disrespected and be very offended.

Cultural Competence: Fundamental Requirements

To provide culturally competent healthcare, providers need to have a culturally sensitive attitude, appropriate cultural knowledge, and flexible enough skills to provide culturally relevant and effective care for the patients of diverse backgrounds. This will allow culturally relevant relations and interactions with patients and families—leading to culturally suitable assessment and care. Physicians, nurses, social workers, and other healthcare providers need to be aware of their own cultural beliefs and biases to be cognizant of their own cultural sensitivity, and to examine the cultural relevance of the healthcare service they provide. This includes assessment and possible modification of the medical culture within which the healthcare is provided. Every patient has a culture, and culture aspects of medical practice need attention whether the patient belong to the minority or the majority.

References

American Anthropology Association (1999) AAA statement on race. American Anthropologist 100(3) 712–713

Baider L, Ever-Hadani P, De Nour AK (1995) The impact of culture on perception of patient-physician satisfaction. Israel Journal of Medical Science, 31(2–3) 179–185

Clements FE (1932) Primitive concepts of disease. American Archaeology and Ethnology (32) 185–252

Currier RL (1966) The hot-cold syndrome and symbol balance in Mexican and Spanish-American folk medicine Ethnology 5(3) 251–263

Good BJ (1977) The heart of what's the matter: The semantics of illness in Iran. Culture, Medicine and Psychiatry 1(1) 25–58

Hoebel EA (1972) Anthropology: The study of man. McGraw-Hill, New York

Stein HF (1993) American medicine as culture. Westview Press, Boulder, CO

Wen JK (1995) Sexual beliefs and problems in contemporary Taiwan. In: Lin TY, Tseng WS, Yeh EK (eds) Chinese Society and Mental Health Oxford University Press, Hong Kong, pp 219–230)

Zuckerman MJ, Guerra LG, Drossman DA, Foland JA, Gregory GG (1996) Healthcare-seeking behaviors related to bowel complaints: Hispanics versus non-Hispanic whites. Digestive Diseases and Sciences 41(1):77–82

Chapter 2
Cultural Competence in Healthcare Specialties

Successful healthcare depends on the teamwork of various professional disciplines, including physicians, nursing, medical technology, physical therapy, social work, nutrition, clinical psychology, and so on. In this chapter, culturally relevant healthcare within several specialties will be discussed.

Care by Physicians

Physicians of all medical specialties need to recognize the importance of cultural issues. To be truly clinically competent, they need to be culturally competent. All patients are influenced by culture, no matter what the ethnic background—be they minorities or majorities. However, particular concern should be directed toward minorities and migrants.

Minorities have been shown to receive inferior healthcare in such areas as referral for cardiac diagnostics and therapeutic procedures, referral for kidney transplants, pain treatment for cancer and fractures, care for pneumonia and heart failure, accessing standard immunizations, and referral for breast cancer and cervical cancer screening. Minorities usually have less health insurance coverage, less healthcare access, more acute and chronic illnesses, and lower life expectancies (Rosa 2006).

The Institute of Medicine—a prestigious advisory organization that is part of the National Academy of Sciences of the United States—has reported on the widespread disparities in healthcare among various minority and cultural groups (Institute of Medicine 2002). It has concluded that these disparities lead to worsened health outcomes, and are unacceptable. It has encouraged the acquisition of cross-cultural skills as one remedy for this problem. This topic has been included in recent texts in family medicine (Taylor 2003) and pediatrics (Behrman, Kliegman & Jenson 2004). Thus, the growing awareness of the need for cultural competence in healthcare has been increasingly recognized, and is being strongly promoted.

Primary care physicians have been found to have less effective communication with ethnic minorities. This causes misunderstandings that are, in turn, associated

W.-S. Tseng and J.M. Streltzer (eds.), *Cultural Competence in Health Care*
© Springer 2008

with noncompliance (Harmsen, Meeuwesen, van Wieringen, Bernsen & Bruijnzeels 2003). Family medicine and internal medicine residents report that they consider cultural competence to be relevant to their clinical work, and that they generally see themselves as fairly sophisticated in cross-cultural communication. If cultural issues cause a problem in communication, however, they tend to blame the problem on patient shortcomings (Shapiro, Hollingshead & Morrison 2003).

Cultural competence training has been recommended for ophthalmologists. Vision impairment disproportionately affects blacks and Hispanics in comparison to whites. Opportunities exist to improve care for diabetic retinopathy, glaucoma, and cataracts in minorities. Culturally appropriate education for physicians and patients offers the best solution to finding strategies to address the care of eye disease in minorities (Wilson & Eezzuduemhoi 2005).

The American Academy of Pediatrics has endorsed the concept of cultural competence as an important part of pediatric practice and a vital social value. It has called for increased diversity in the workforce and cultural education and training from medical school through ongoing CME activities (American Academy of Pediatrics Committee on Pediatric Workforce 2004).

A recent prospective study evaluated the treatment of asthma in children in managed Medicaid practice sites in three states. It found that policies designed to promote cultural competence were a main factor in predicting higher quality asthma care (Lieu, Finkelstein, Lozano, Capra, Chi, Jensvold, Quesenberry & Farber 2004). In a study of informed consent, it was shown that the content and quality of physician communication differed depending on parents' ethnicity, perhaps reflecting physician attitudes toward the ethnicity (Simon & Kodish 2005).

Surbone (2006) has called for culturally competent cancer care, which is important not only at the level of the healthcare provider, but also at the systems and organizational levels. He defines culturally competent cancer care as being "based on knowledge of the notion of culture; on awareness of possible biases and prejudices related to stereotyping, racism, classism, sexism; on nurturing appreciation for differences in healthcare values; and on fostering the attitudes of humility, empathy, curiosity, respect, sensitivity and awareness" (Surbone 2006).

Obstetrics and gynecology (OB-GYN) is a special field of medicine that only concerns health issues specific to women—usually related to the reproductive organs. In many countries, OB-GYN doctors are predominately male. This was originally also true in the United States (Haar, Halitsky & Stricker 1975). Now, however, the majority of OB-GYN residents in training are women, in conjunction with a cultural shift in the attitudes of women patients. Between 1999 and 2003, the number of male graduates of OB-GYN training programs decreased 31.3 percent, while female graduates increased 18.2 percent. In a typical study, 53 percent of women stated they would prefer a female gynecologist, 10 percent would prefer a male, and 37 percent had no preference. Most women, however, found that other factors were more important than the gender of their physician, including competence, bedside manner, and experience (Plunkett, Kohlip & Milad 2002). As women doctors increasingly take care of women patients, there is concern that the productivity of these physicians will be less due to socioeconomic reasons, such as their own need to give birth and raise children. It is estimated that the productivity of female OB-GYN doctors will be 85 percent that of males, and that this will lead to, or exacerbate, future physician shortages (Pearse 2001). There is also concern about a decline in the number of medical students choosing OB-GYN as a specialty, partly because of the hard work, the need of availability for night deliveries, and the high cost for medical malpractice insurance for this specialty. Some OB-GYN doctors have been sued two decades after the delivery of a baby. Thus, the looming shortage reflects not only medical issues, but also social and cultural matters.

Residency training programs in all specialties are increasingly including cultural competence in their curricula. In 2003, 50.7 percent of programs provided opportunities for developing cultural competence—a rapid and substantial increase from 2000 when the percentage was 35.7 percent (Brotherton, Rockey & Etzel 2004). In pediatrics, cultural competence and antiracism training appears to be not only well-received, but effective in facilitating quality care (Webb & Sergison 2004). A survey of residents receiving training in cultural competence, however, found that although the issue was presented to them as being important, little time was actually allotted to cross-cultural issues, nor was there much in the way of training, formal evaluation, or role modeling (Weissman, Betancourt, Campbell, Park, Kim, Clarridge, Blumenthal, Lee & Maina 2005).

Among medical school faculty however, minorities are underrepresented. In 2003, 75 percent of fulltime faculty members were white, 5.8 percent were African-American, and only 3 percent were Hispanic. The proportion of underrepresented minority faculty has not increased from 1998 to 2003 (Barzansky 2003). This is a significant issue because access to and interaction with faculty and peers from different cultural groups will usually enhance cultural sensitivity.

Among medical schools with cross-cultural education curricula, considerable variation has been found. Themes included the doctor-patient relationship, racism, socioeconomic status, and specific information about the ethnic communities being served (Peña Dolhun, Muñoz & Grumbach 2003). Some programs recommend or utilize immersion programs and even language training to provide cross-cultural skills.

Many medical schools have adopted the LEARN model (Berlin & Fowkes Jr. 1983). This consists of the following objectives:

L - Listen to your patient from his or her cultural perspective
E - Explain your reasons for asking for personal information
A - Acknowledge your patient's concerns
R - Recommend a course of action
N - Negotiate a plan that takes into consideration your patient's cultural norms and personal lifestyles

A more recently developed mnemonic to provide training is the CRASH course in cultural competency. CRASH designates certain components considered essential to culturally competent healthcare: consider Culture, show Respect, Assess/ Affirm differences, show Sensitivity and Self-awareness, and do it all with Humility (Rust, Kondwani, Martinez, Dansie, Wong, Fry-Johnson, Woody, Daniels, Herbert-Carter, Aponte & Strothers 2006).

After an extensive review of research relevant to cultural competence, Rosa (2006) concluded that while there was little in the way of outcome studies on the effect of cultural competence on patient health, there was good evidence that cultural competence improved patient-physician communication and interaction, and is necessary for high-quality patient care.

Care by Nurses

Cultural competence is recognized as a key component of nursing care. Cultural competence in nursing has been comprehensively defined as "an ongoing process with the goal of achieving the ability to work effectively with culturally diverse groups and communities with a detailed awareness, specific knowledge, refined skills and personal and professional respect for cultural attributes, both differences and similarities" (Suh 2004). The concept of *transcultural nursing* has been advocated by nurses for many decades (Leininger & McFarland 2002, p. 3–37; Giger & Davidhizar 1999, pp.3–19). This involves caring for patients who have different ethnic/cultural backgrounds from their nurses, and is derived from the clinical experiences with patients of various ethnic/cultural groups in multiethnic societies (Callister 2005; Cioffi 2005). Cultural competence in nursing care is particularly emphasized by community and public health nurses through their encounters with clients from distinctly different sociocultural settings (Degazon 2004). Learning to inquire into an individual's personal interpretations of life's world experiences rather than relying on catalogs of cultural attributes and stereotypes has been shown to increase nurses' confidence in providing a more culturally competent, higher quality of patient care (Kleiman 2006). Recruitment and training of culturally diverse nursing practitioners is considered an important objective in achieving the goal of culturally competent nursing care (Pacquiao 2007).

General Issues

The Role and Status of Nurses

The role, status, and function of nurses vary in different societies. They are basically shaped by the social culture and medical culture operating in a given society at a particular time. For example, in many Asian societies, physicians have relatively complete authority in administrating inpatient services, and nurses have only subordinate status and supplementary roles in providing nursing care. In many European-American societies, on the other hand, nurses play major roles in administrating services in the inpatient unit, while physicians only provide medical treatment.

The different role and status of nurses in different cultures is exemplified by the situation in Thailand. There, nurses are discouraged from thinking and acting independently. Thus, nurses trained in Thailand are not suited to work in Western settings (Ekintumas 1999).

Relations with Physicians

In many countries, most physicians are male and most nurses are female. As a result, physician-nurse relationships are subject to the male-female gender relationships defined in society. In Japan, for example, where men still generally have a higher status than women, nurses are expected to bow to physicians when they meet them. Nurses are expected to play only supplementary and subordinate roles under physicians (Long 1984). In the United States, however, this hierarchy is less obvious, and nurses and physicians relate to each other more or less in a spirit of equality and democracy, while retaining their own areas of expertise.

Relations with Patients

In general, nurses have a great deal of direct contact with patients, providing care and maintaining a close relationship. This is particularly true in a society where physicians play rather authoritative roles in their relations with patients. Physicians' interactions with patients are relatively minimal and professional distance is maintained. In this situation, patients feel that nurses are the staff with whom they can communicate and to whom they can relate. Questions or concerns are addressed to the nurses, rather than the physicians. Nurses play the role of intermediary between physicians and patients and their families (see Chapter 1).

Special Issues Relating to Nursing Care

Assessment and Judgment of the Patient's Behavior

In addition to general medical professional competency, nurses need to develop cultural competency in their care of medical patients in the same way as physicians. Competent nursing practice must include being able to negotiate care in an encounter where at least some of the beliefs, values, attitudes and experiences of the nurse and patient differ. It is appropriate for nurses to acquire specific knowledge about what possible aspects of a client's ethnic identity and cultural background may have a bearing on healthcare (Culley 2001). Cultural competence also includes learning how to observe and understand the patients', as well as their families', behavior from a cultural standpoint, so that proper assessment can be made and relevant care can be provided.

Matters Related to Nurturing and Independence

Even though nurturance for ill or disabled patients is a basic part of nursing care, careful consideration needs to be given to what nurturing care means for a given patient and what nurturance needs to be provided. Patients often need to be encouraged to care for themselves for the sake of faster rehabilitation. Healthcare professionals should generally be careful not to deprive patients of the opportunity of self-healing and self-recovery. However, to what extent nurturing care is appropriate is a matter of not only professional, but also sociocultural, judgement and definition. A culturally competent nurse will sensitively reveal what is expected from patients and their families, tailoring explanations and education to the individual needs of the patient.

Care by Social Workers

The primary work of the medical social worker involves assisting the family to determine how to provide care for the patient and to help the patient and family utilize the resources of support that exist in the community or social system. The social worker performs the service as an adjunct to the physician or other healthcare providers, or independently. Overall, service is heavily focused on the family, community, and social system at large. The concept of, and the need for, culturally relevant social work has been recognized for some time (Ewalt, Freeman, Kirk & Poole 1996; Triseliotis 1986). All accredited schools of social work include cultural diversity in their curriculum (Boyle & Springer 2001).

Common Issues

Working with Family

Pediatricians typically work with parents when treating a child, and geriatricians often involve adult children or a spouse when treating an elderly person. When treating young and middle-aged adults, however, modern physicians with Western backgrounds seldom consider the need to involve family members. This stems from the Western physician's basic philosophical attitude that respects an individual's autonomy.

However, this is not necessarily the best practice from a cultural perspective. For many cultures, family ties and interpersonal relationships are so tight that an individual seldom functions by him or herself. If a person becomes sick, he or she may be accompanied by parents, spouse, and/or children, and visited by a group of relatives or friends. This is a culture-derived custom. A social worker can take the opportunity to involve family members whenever they are available. Providing support to the family will support the patient (Tseng & Hsu 1991). On the other hand, a recent study of family support in both blacks and whites found that, contrary to earlier reports, blacks did not enjoy greater family support. The study cautioned practitioners not to assume that blacks have stronger family support systems (Griffin, Amodeo, Clay, Fassler & Ellis 2006).

Working with the Community

Communities differ in terms of socioeconomic status, medical facilities and systems, and the ethnic and cultural backgrounds of its members. To maximally utilize the support resources available in the community or society at large, it is necessary for the social worker to be familiar with the nature, structure, and system of the community and society. In addition, it is also important that they know the patient's and the family's knowledge, attitudes, and ability to utilize existing social support systems—including social welfare and other services. This is particularly true for foreigners or new immigrants who are unfamiliar with many aspects of the host society that may be quite different from their home societies. Patients or their families may have very different attitudes toward public support systems, such as welfare. Some do not hesitate to accept social welfare, while others tend to avoid such assistance, considering it shameful. Social-work interventions have successfully used culture-based techniques, and such techniques can sometimes be adapted for use in other communities (Hurdle 2002).

Special Functions and Services

Social workers at large in a community are often involved directly or indirectly in various health-related services. These may include mental health services relating to child protection. If these services involve clients of diverse ethnic or racial backgrounds—particularly with communication problems due to language or conceptual issues—special care is warranted. For example, taking small (abused) children away from their (abusing) parents and placing them in foster homes for the purpose of *protection* is an entirely Western concept, and a practice that has never been heard of or practiced in many Eastern societies, where the togetherness of the family is incontrovertibly valued and respected. To what extent parents are allowed or expected to carry out physical discipline of their children varies greatly among different cultures. To what extent parents can acceptably have physical contact with their small children is also different in various societies. Therefore, workers involved with the assessment of child abuse, either physical or sexual, need to consider cultural norms in working with and supporting these families. Ideally, they can help families understand and adapt to new cultural norms, if necessary.

Care by Physical Therapists

The Concept of Physical Therapy

Contemporary medical practice encourages rapid physical mobilization after medical and surgical illness—such as myocardial infarction and total hip replacement—

and physical therapy is often an important part of rehabilitation. Such a concept may not be congruent with the cultural concepts held by some people, however, who believe that rest is the best way to recuperate from their illness. Saving energy is a traditional folk concept to help the body recover and regain health. If cultural issues are suspected, the physical therapist must not assume that patients (as well as families) automatically understand the usefulness of physical activity to facilitate recovery.

Cultural Aspects of Physical Contact

To perform physical therapy, the therapist usually needs to have physical contact with the patient. The spatial distance between the therapist and the patient is also quite close even when contact is not being made. Interpersonal distance and allowable physical contact (particularly between genders) are strongly determined by cultural norms. Awareness of this issue allows the therapist to sensitively manage the needed contact. This, of course, applies to all healthcare providers who need to have close physical contact with the patient (see Chapter 3: The Physical Examination).

Dietary

The nutritionist, often an important member of the healthcare team, plays a significant role for patients with special dietary needs due to their medical conditions, such as diabetes, kidney disorders, hypertension, gout, and others. In addition to educating patients and families how to prepare and consume certain food from a medical perspective, nutritionists should be able to adjust diets to fulfill cultural needs.

Cultural Aspects of Food

Food is more than just a source of nutrition. Food plays many roles and is deeply embedded in the social, religious, and economic aspects of everyday life. Food carries with it range of symbolic meanings—both expressing and creating the relationships between man and man, between man and his deities, and between man and the natural environment. Food is an essential part of the way that all societies organize themselves and view the world (Helman 2000, p. 32). In essence, food is a major part of a culture.

Each culture defines which substances are edible and which are not, leaving out concerns about nutritional value (Helman, 2000, pp. 33–34). For instance, orthodox Hindus are forbidden to kill or eat any animal, particularly the cow. Milk and its products may be consumed because they do not involve taking an animal's life. Fish are infrequently eaten. For Muslims, neither pork nor any pig products may be eaten. The only meat permitted is that from cloven-hoofed animals that chew their cud, and they must be ritually slaughtered (*halal*). Only fish that have fins and scales may be eaten, so shellfish, shark, and eels are therefore forbidden. For Jews (similarly to Muslims), all pig products are forbidden, and only animals that chew their cud, have cloven hooves, and have been ritually slaughtered are *kosher* and may be eaten. Furthermore, meat and milk dishes are never mixed within the same meal. Believers of Buddhism consider all living beings that can move around as having a soul, and the killing of them is forbidden. Accordingly, they are vegetarian and do not eat meat or even seafood. Of course, many people's preference for a vegetarian diet is unrelated to any religious belief.

The division of all foodstuffs into two groups—either *hot* or *cold*—is a feature of many cultures in the Islamic world, the Indian subcontinent, Latin America, and Eastern Asia. In all these cultures, this binary system of classification of food is a part of the overall concepts of health, the environment, and the universe. What food is actually classified as hot or cold may vary from culture to culture, based on local history and cultural factors.

People's food preferences are a result of mixed reasons, namely, physiological tolerance, past experiences, psychological interpretations, and religion-related beliefs. It is not only the food preference, but the manner in which food is prepared or cooked, that is determined by cultural tradition.

In a study of Hispanics and African-Americans in Detroit, Michigan, greater fruit and vegetable consumption was associated with people who had more than a high school education and more advanced age among Hispanics, and with more exercise and older age among African Americans. Lower fruit and vegetable consumption was associated with people who had less education, smoked, and were male among African Americans. By learning about health behaviors in high-risk communities, interventions and policies for reducing racial and ethnic disparities in healthcare can be more effectively planned (Kieffer, Sinco, Rafferty, Spencer, Palmisano, Watt & Heisler 2006).

References

American Academy of Pediatrics Committee on Pediatric Workforce (2004) Ensuring culturally effective pediatric care: Implications for education and health policy. Pediatrics 114:1677–1685

Barzansky B (2003) Educational programs in US medical schools 2002–2003. JAMA 290:1190–1196

Behrman RE, Kliegman RM, Jenson HB (2004) Nelson Textbook of Pediatrics, 17th edn. Saunders, Philadelphia

Berlin, E.A. & Fowkes, W.C. Jr. (1983). A teaching framework for cross-cultural health care: Application in family practice, *Western Journal of Medicine*. 139, 934–938.

Boyle DP, Springer A (2001) Toward a cultural competence measure for social work with specific populations. Journal of Ethnic and Cultural Diversity in Social Work 9:53–71

Brotherton SE, Rockey PH, Etzel SI (2004) US graduate medical education, 2003–2004. JAMA 292:1032–7

Callister LC (2005) What has the literature taught us about culturally competent care of women and children. MCN: American Journal of Maternal Child Nursing 30:380–388

Cioffi J (2005) Nurses' experience of caring for culturally diverse patients in an acute care setting. Contemporary Nurse 20:78–86

Culley L (2001) Nursing, culture and competence. In: Culley L, Dyson S (eds) Ethnicity and Nursing Practice Palgrave, New York, pp 109–127

Degazon CE (2004) Cultural diversity and community-oriented nursing practice. In: Stanhope M, Lancaster J (eds) Community and Public Health Nursing, 6th edn Mosby, St. Louis, Missouri, pp 148–169

Ekintumas D (1999) Nursing in Thailand: Western concepts vs Thai tradition. International Nursing Review 46:55–7

Ewalt PL, Freeman EM, Kirk SA, Poole DL (eds) (1996) Multicultural Issues in Social Work. NASW (National Association of Social Workers) Press, Washington, D.C.

Giger JN, Davidhizar RE (eds) (1999) Transcultural Nursing: Assessment & Intervention, 3rd edn. Mosby, St. Louis, Missouri

Griffin ML, Amodeo M, Clay C, Fassler I, Ellis MA (2006) Racial differences in social support: Kin versus friends. American Journal of Orthopsychiatry 76:374–80

Haar E, Halitsky V, Stricker G (1975) Factors related to the preference for a female gynecologist. Medical Care 13:782–90

Harmsen H, Meeuwesen L, van Wieringen J, Bernsen R Bruijnzeels M (2003) When cultures meet in general practice: Intercultural differences between GPs and parents of child patients. Patient Education and Counseling 51:99–106

Helman CG (2000) Culture, Health and Illness, 4th Edn. Butterworth-Heinemann, Oxford, pp 32–49

Hurdle DE (2002) Native Hawaiian traditional healing: culturally based interventions for social work practice. Social Work 47:183–92

Institute of Medicine (2002) Unequal Treatment: Confronting Racial and Ethnic Disparities in Healthcare. National Academy Press, Washington D.C.

Kieffer EC, Sinco BR, Rafferty A, Spencer MS, Palmisano G, Watt EE, Heisler M (2006) Chronic disease-related behaviors and health among African Americans and Hispanics in the REACH Detroit 2010 communities, Michigan, and the United States. Health Promotion Practice 7(3 Suppl):256S–264S

Kleiman S (2006) Discovering cultural aspects of nurse-patient relationships. Journal of Cultural Diversity 13:83–6

Leininger M McFarland MR (eds) (2002) Transcultural Nursing: Concepts, Ttheories, Research and Practice. 3rd edn. McGraw-Hill, New York

Lieu TA, Finkelstein JA, Lozano P, Capra AM, Chi FW, Jensvold N, Quesenberry CP, Farber HJ (2004) Cultural competence policies and other predictors of asthma care quality for Medicaid-insured children. Pediatrics 114:102–110

Long SO (1984) The sociocultural context of nursing in Japan. Culture, Medicine and Psychiatry 8:141–163

Pacquiao D (2007) The relationship between cultural competence education and increasing diversity in nursing schools and practice settings. Journal of Transcultural Nursing 18 (Suppl 1):28S–37S

Pearse W.H, Haffner WH, Primack A (2001) Effect of gender on the obstetric-gynecologic work force. Obstetrics and Gynecology 97:794–797

Peña Dolhun E, Muñoz C, Grumbach K (2003) Cross-cultural education in U.S. medical schools: Development of an assessment tool. Academic Medicine 78:615–622.

Plunkett BA, Kohlip P,, Milad HP (2002) The importance of physician gender in the selection of an obstritician or a gynecologist. American Journal of Obstetrics and Gynecology 186:926–928

Rosa UW (2006) Impact of cultural competence on medical care: Where are we today? Clinics in Chest Medicine 27:395–9

Rust G, Kondwani K, Martinez R, Dansie R, Wong W, Fry-Johnson Y, Woody Rdel M, Daniels EJ, Herbert-Carter J, Aponte L, Strothers H (2006) A crash-course in cultural competence. Ethnicity and Disease 16(2 Suppl 3):S3-29–36

Shapiro J, Hollingshead J, Morrison E (2003) Self-perceived attitudes and skills of cultural competence: A comparison of family medicine and internal medicine residents. Medical Teacher 25:327–329

Simon CM, Kodish ED (2005) Step into my zapatos, doc: Understanding and reducing communication disparities in the multicultural informed consent setting. Perspectives in Biology and Medicine 48(1 Suppl):S139–149

Suh EE (2004) The model of cultural competence through an evolutionary concept analysis. Journal of Transcultural Nursing 15:93–102

Surbone A (2006) Cultural aspects of communication in cancer care. Recent Results in Cancer Research, 168:91–104

Taylor RB (ed) (2003) *Family medicine: Principles and practice*. Springer, New York

Triseliotis J (1986) Transcultural social work. In: Cox J (ed) Transcultural Psychiatry Croom Helm, London, pp196–217

Tseng WS, Hsu J (1991) *Culture and family: Problems and therapy*. The Haworth Press, New York

Weissman JS, Betancourt J, Campbell EG, Park ER, Kim M, Clarridge B, Blumenthal D, Lee KC, Maina AW (2005) Resident physicians' preparedness to provide cross-cultural care. JAMA 294:1058–1067

Wilson MR Eezzuduemhoi DR (2005) Ophthalmologic disorders in minority populations. Medical Clinics of North America 89:795–804

Chapter 3
Culture and Clinical Assessment

To perform a competent, relevant, and thorough assessment of a patient, cultural issues must be taken into account. The components of clinical assessment, including observation of the patient, history-taking, physical examination, and laboratory testing, all may be influenced by cultural factors. The cultural issues are most obvious if the patient has a distinctly different background from the healthcare provider. The patient may have very different beliefs and understanding of a particular illness. Symptoms and complaints related to a given condition may be presented very differently, and the patient's attitude about being examined and tested may vary substantially. If the patient speaks a different language from that of the clinician, an interpreter will be needed for translation. This involves special considerations and skills on the part of both the interpreter and the clinician.

Presentation of Problems

In a manner that can be quite subtle, a patient's style of presenting complaints is influenced by cultural factors. In general, how presenting problems and their symptoms are described is subject to the patient's educational level, medical knowledge, and motivation for treatment, as well as their culturally patterned modes of problem presentation.

"I feel my heart is empty!", "There is a fire elevation within my chest!", and "I am concerned that my semen is leaking from my urine!" are some examples of culturally flavored symptom presentations that may be observed among various ethnic groups in Asia or South Asia. Clearly semantic factors are involved, but these presentations also reflect folk concepts of illness. For instance, Chinese people may use *empty heart* or *injured heart* to describe a depressed mood to a healthcare professional without insinuating any relation to cardiac symptoms. An American may talk of being *brokenhearted*, but this reflects feelings of disappointment, usually communicated to a confidant in a social context, rather than to communicate medical concerns. A Korean person may complain of a *fire elevation* (within the body) to indicate excessive fire elements, which refer to emotionally upsetting conditions. When an Eastern Indian man is concerned that his semen might be leaking from his urine, and asks for an examination of his urine, he is using a culture-patterned concept and expression regarding an illness called *dhat* (also known by cultural psychiatrists as *spermatorrhea*) to indicate that he has anxieties about some issue. A culturally sensitive physician will try to understand the symbolic meaning behind what is said rather than taking the complaint literally.

Whether or not a patient focuses more on somatic symptoms when presenting psychological problems is influenced by his understanding of the suffering and his motivation for seeking care. It is also shaped by cultural influences. A depressed patient, for example, may complain that his or her mood is *down*—feeling sad, miserable and pessimistic, with loss of interest in life. The patient is using a psychological framework and thus presents the *psychological* aspects of depression. This presentation of symptoms is determined by social assumptions and a cultural attitude that it is acceptable to complain about one's emotions and feelings, even when they are negative ones. The common expectation is that when a person is depressed, medical attention is appropriate. There is medication for depression. There is a need to talk to someone to get help. Therefore, it will be much easier for the healthcare provider to understand that the patient is suffering from depression emotionally and provide proper care accordingly. In contrast, some patients may choose to present the somatic aspects of depression. They may complain about loss of appetite, feeling tired, having no energy, headache, or back pain, difficulty sleeping, and so on. This patient may believe that depression is a common problem (therefore there is no point in asking for help); that it is a sign of weakness (and it is better not to complain to others about personal weakness); that it is proper and legitimate to complain of somatic symptoms to physicians and other healthcare providers (who are concerned about the body); and that it is a useful and effective way to get attention from others and family members (rather than complain about sadness). The initial presentation of somatic complaints can be a culturally patterned style of relating to healthcare providers even though the real emotional problems may be described later. Quite a dramatic example of this is the Chinese patient who makes somatically oriented complaints about *empty heart* or *weak heart, weak kidneys* or *insufficient kidneys, elevated liver fire*, or *irritated spleen*. These complaints may sound odd to contemporary, educated healthcare providers, and it is helpful to know that they simply reflect the fact that the patient is using cultural idioms from traditional Chinese medicine, which are characterized by the organ-based conceptions of psychopathology.

Understanding Patient's Medical Knowledge

A patient's understanding of, and attitude toward, certain medical disorders may influence the way they present problems, thus affecting clinical assessment. Cultural factors are often important in this regard. Matsumoto, Pun, Nakatani, Kadowaki, Weissman, McCarter, Fletcher, and Takeuchi (1995) compared first- and second-generation Japanese-American women in San Francisco concerning their attitudes and beliefs about osteoporosis. First-generation Japanese-American women attributed osteoporosis to fate or luck. Second-generation women were much more aware of the contributions of diet and other risk factors, and therefore potentially more amenable to behavior modification to reduce osteoporosis.

Carpenter and Colwell (1995) pointed out that Latino women are at significantly greater risk of death from cancer than Caucasian women in the United States due to a lack of knowledge regarding cancer, lack of access to cancer-screening services, and feelings of fatalism. From their survey of Mexican-American women living in Texas, they reported that increased knowledge is associated with increased self-efficacy for cancer screening.

As a part of a cancer-prevention program aimed at minority and disadvantaged urban women, the cancer beliefs, knowledge, and behaviors of home-health attendants in the Bronx, New York City were assessed by Morgan, Park, and Cortes (1995). They found that nearly 60 percent of Hispanic women surveyed did not know what cervical cancer was, and nearly 60 percent believed that surgery causes cancer to spread.

Dancy (1996) surveyed African-American women of different ages and educational levels in Chicago to compare their knowledge and attitudes on AIDS. It was found that educational level influenced knowledge about AIDS, whereas age did not influence knowledge about AIDS but did influence attitudes and sexual behavior. This illustrated that African-Americans are not a homogeneous group in terms of their understanding of, and reaction to, a specific medical disorder. Age and educational levels are among the variables attributed to differences within the same ethnic groups.

Hodes and Teferedegne (1996) interviewed Ethiopian Jews (Falashas) about the cause of certain medical conditions. They found that interviewees thought epilepsy was caused by spirits and recommended inhaling smoke as a treatment. Prolonged labor was due to evil spirits, and miscarriages were due to exposure to sun or cold. Less than 20 percent of interviewees were able to link malaria to mosquito bite transmission.

These studies illustrate that the medical knowledge of patients may vary significantly, and may shape their health concerns, help-seeking patterns, and style of presenting complaints, and thus influence the process and outcome of medical assessment.

History Taking

The process of gathering medical information from the patient is subject to various factors. It depends on the patient's age, personality, intelligence, cognitive style, ability to communicate, and motivation for seeking help. The process is also influenced by the patient's understanding of the illness, which involves both medical knowledge and idiosyncratic beliefs. Therefore, cultural factors will influence the patient's presentation of problems.

Clinicians are typically trained to take down a straightforward medical history, asking about the chief complaint, the history of present illness, pertinent past medical history, and family history. A premium is placed on obtaining the needed information within a limited timeframe. This is particularly true in an emergency room or busy outpatient settings. This style of history taking and assessment, however, may not work well for people of some cultures. It may be important to *talk story* for a while before moving into the exploration of serious medical problems. *Talk story* is a term used by people in Hawaii, meaning to chat and converse for socialization. Asking a patient where they live, talking about relatives, neighbors, the weather, food, and so forth, can sometimes help establish rapport. This process may seem like wasting time, but it will be a culturally appropriate way to ultimately obtain the important medical information in the most effective, and indeed efficient, manner. Rushing to inquire into sensitive medical problems may not get desirable results from patients who need to first establish a comfortable and trusting relationship with the healthcare provider. In contrast, if the healthcare provider spends too much time socializing by *talking story* with a patient or family whose culture emphasizes efficiency and practicality, they may feel that the healthcare provider is not sure how to approach the medical matter and is indeed wasting time *chatting*.

Before inquiring about sensitive subjects, it is generally better to start with easy subjects (such as appetite, pain, or discomfort), and gradually approach the more sensitive matters (such as menstruation, sexual desire, or sexual functioning). It is always helpful to explain why healthcare providers need to ask about *private* matters, and provide assurance that the information obtained will be kept confidential for medical purposes only.

When the patient and the care provider are of different genders, extra caution is needed. This is particularly true for patients brought up in a culture with a distinct boundary between man and woman. When a female physician or care provider asks a male patient about his sexual life, he may feel offended, defensive, or embarrassed because of a culturally-based belief that men should be assumed to be sexually competent with women. It is therefore insulting or embarrassing to have this subject explored by a female.

There are wide cultural variations influencing a female's response to inquiries about sexual issues from a male healthcare provider. In some cultures, there are such strong prohibitions against women sharing such information with men that this carries over even into the medical setting. At times, it may be helpful to ask the assistance of care providers of the same gender as the patient to explore such sensitive and *private* matters. For female patients, the presence of a husband, mother, or elder sister may ease the situation.

Doctor-Patient Relationship

Beyond the matter of communication between the doctor or other healthcare provider and the patient, is how the relationship between them will determine the richness and validity of information gathering and influence the prescribed therapy. If a patient is coming from a culture that emphasizes hierarchy and stresses respect for authority, that patient's attitude and behavior toward authority figures may dominate the relationship with the doctor, who is seen as a person representing authority. The following case illustrates how the patient's attitude toward authority shaped his relationship with the physician, which in turn, resulted in problems in the process of treatment.

A 62-year old, first generation, Filipino-American male patient was seen by a American doctor for a checkup. After the initial visit, the patient's blood pressure was found to be 160/104, so the physician prescribed an antihypertensive medicine for him. At the follow-up visit, the patient's blood pressure was still high: 162/98. The doctor asked the patient: "Did you take the medication that I prescribed for you?" "Yes, doctor!" answered the patient. The doctor increased the dose, and asked the patient to return the next week for follow-up. When the patient came back, the doctor found the patient's blood pressure was still very high. The doctor asked the patient again: "Are you taking the medication that I prescribed for you?" "Yes, doctor!" answered the patient again. The doctor then questioned the patient's wife, who had been present but silent at each visit. She informed the doctor that the patient stopped taking the medication after the very first dose, because it made him feel *dizzy*. He dared not to tell the doctor that he did not like the medicine prescribed for him, and thus kept saying "Yes, doctor!" obediently when he was asked by the physician whether he was taking the medication as prescribed. This illustrates how the patient is relating to the physician and responding to the physician's inquiry by deferring to authority (with respect and no opposition), as he was raised to do in his culture (Streltzer 2004).

The Use of Interpreters

When the patient or family does not share the same language as the physician, nurse, social worker, or other healthcare provider, it becomes necessary to use language interpreters for assessment and care. An important issue is who is going to be used as an interpreter. In general, family members have the advantage of knowing the patient's concerns and background, but they may make incorrect assumptions. Furthermore, the patient may not want the family to know of issues he or she prefers to be kept in confidence. It is particularly not a good idea to ask younger children to serve as the interpreter for a parent, even though in immigrant families children usually learn the language of the host society faster than their parents. The parent not only may be reluctant to share certain problems, but this also may contribute to a reversal of the authority aspects of the parent-child relationship.

Professional interpreters are generally preferred, if possible. It is particularly desirable that the professional interpreter have some medical knowledge in addition to the familiarity and fluency of the language involved. Whether the interpreter belongs to the same ethnic group of the patient, and is of the same gender or age background, are some of the issues that need to be considered as well. For patients from very conservative cultures, the use of an interpreter of the gender opposite that of the patient may limit the information that can be obtained.

If a language and behavior are going to be understood correctly, and be meaningful, consideration of the cross-cultural equivalence and validity of the translation is necessary (Tseng 2001, pp. 477–478). For instance, simply translating the complaint of *fire elevation within my chest!* or *empty heart* literally will be not enough. The culturally competent translator should be able to properly interpret that these statements mean: *full of so much anger and resentment that I'm feeling a fire sensation rising within me*, or *depressed in such a way that the heart feels empty*, respectively.

Technical errors potentially made by interpreters include deletion or omission of information, exaggeration or addition of information, and inaccurate translation of words or concepts—not only from the semantic point of view, but also from a cultural perspective (Lee 1997). In contrast to this, mistakes often made by clinicians are failure to work closely with the interpreter as a partner, failure to interact directly with the patient (only with the interpreter), and an inability to detect paralinguistic or nonverbal behavior. In essence, healthcare providers need training in how to use interpreters properly and effectively (Luk 2006).

Subjects Likely to be Culturally Influenced

Care of Children

Because children are immature and vulnerable, both physically and mentally, they are dependent upon their adult caretakers—usually the parents—for survival. In the early stages of language and cognition development, young children are not yet capable of clear communication about the nature of their condition. Healthcare providers must rely on the parent(s) or parent substitute(s) to describe the problems the children are suffering. If the adults have their own biases or folk interpretations of the children's medical problems, their description and management of the child's illness may be shaped by these beliefs and understandings.

The following example, described by Fernandez, South-Paul, and Matheny (2003, p. 21), illustrates how parents can view the medical problems in a widely different way from that of the clinicians. A women who recently moved to Los Angeles from central Mexico brought her 11-month old child to the clinic with symptoms of diarrhea and signs of mild dehydration. Through the interpreter, the mother complained to the clinician that the child had *mollera caida* (literally, *fallen fontanelle*). Her method of treatment was to place salt on spots, and give the child *manzanilla* (chamomile) tea. The clinician, on the other hand, was concerned about the etiology of the diarrhea and wanted to initiate oral rehydration.

The following case demonstrates a similar point. A young child was brought to see a pediatrician by the mother who had recently migrated from Vietnam to the United States. The mother, using a coin, scratched the child's abdomen, causing numerous bruises. The American pediatrician suspected child abuse as the cause of the lesions. A child protection agency was about to be contacted, until a nurse of Asian background intervened. She informed the doctor that scratching the skin was an Asian folk remedy thought to help heal a feverish child. Traditional Asian medicine interprets a fever as the result of excessive yang elements in the body. Scratching and bruising the skin helps the patient expel the excessive yang from the body.

Pregnancy, Childbirth, and Postpartum Care

Pregnancy and giving birth are major events that have substantial cultural significance and are impacted by cultural beliefs. Woollet, Dosanjh, Nicolson, Marshall, Djhanbakhch, and Hadlow (1995) compared the ideas and experiences of pregnancy and childbirth of Asian and non-Asian women in east London. Although Asian women demonstrated a strong commitment to accessing Western maternity care, they continued to follow traditional cultural practices such as observing a special diet in pregnancy and following restrictions on certain activities in the post-partum period. Both parents, as well the grandparents, tended to be more concerned with the gender of the child.

In some ethnic groups, great attention is paid to post-partum care. Traditional Chinese beliefs require a woman to observe one month of confinement after giving birth. She is not allowed to go outside of her house, to consume cold foods (such as fruits), to bathe, or even wash her hair. The new mother is supposed to eat more hot foods (such as chicken cooked with sesame oil and ginger). These were old customs that may have originated to prevent post-partum infection yet are still faithfully observed by some women. In Micronesia, a traditional pregnancy custom requires the wife to return to her family of origin once she discovers she is pregnant. She does not return to live with her husband until her child is old enough to hold his breath under water or to jump across a ditch, activities that ensure the greater likelihood of the child's survival.

Breast-feeding is a very natural way to feed a newborn baby. Despite the widely acknowledged evidence supporting the medical benefits of breast-feeding (such as fewer childhood infections and allergies), however, the prevalence and duration of breast-feeding in Western countries remains relatively low. This may be due to the availability of baby formula or time demands on a working mom. Rodriguez-Garcia and Frazier (1995) point out that the cultural notion of the female breast as a primarily sexual object places the act of breast-feeding in a controversial light and can be one of the most influential factors in a woman's decision not to breast-feed.

Breast Cancer

The varying degrees to which female breasts have a sexual role in different cultures may influence the patient's understanding of the causes of breast cancer. Chavez,

Hubbell, McMullin, Martinez, and Mishra (1995) interviewed Salvadoran immigrants, Mexican immigrants, Chicanas, and Anglo-Americans in California concerning attitudes toward risk factors for breast cancer. They found two broad cultural models. The Anglo-American model emphasized family history and age as risk factors. The Latin model associated breast trauma and *bad* behaviors (such as alcohol and illegal drug use) as risk factors for breast cancer. A subsequent investigation by Hubbell, Chavez, Mishra, and Valdez (1996) in California found that Latinas were more likely than Anglo-American women to believe that factors such as breast trauma (71% vs. 39%) and breast fondling (27% vs. 6%) increased the risk of breast cancer. The investigators concluded that Latinas' beliefs about breast cancer may reflect the moral framework within which they interpret diseases.

Sexual Orientation and Behavior

This is usually a sensitive subject to explore—even for medical reasons—for people of any cultural background, but it is particularly so for people from conservative cultures. For many contemporary Westerners, it may be easy to talk about sexual orientation and even sexual behavior. The words *sexual intercourse* are easily used nowadays. However, it is rather difficult and even taboo for people from some cultures. *Intimacy between husband and wife* or *bedroom business* may be used instead.

Menstruation and Menopause

Although menstruation and menopause are biological phenomena, these are sex-related subjects. *Monthly cycle*, or *women's cycle* (or *business*), are some of the terms used to avoid the embarrassing feeling associated with the word of *menstruation*. Among Chinese female adolescents in Taiwan, the created term of *number one* is used to avoid mentioning menstruation.

Regarding menopause, the intensity of menopausal symptoms varies among ethnic or racial groups (Tseng 2001). This may be due partially to diet, with a recent study revealing that Asian women may experience fewer hot flashes because of estrogen derived from soybean products in their meals. To what extent sexual attitudes contribute to emotional adjustment or attitudes toward menopause is a subject that requires future investigation. It is a relatively easy subject to bring up with women, particularly by women clinicians, but it may be embarrassing for women of conservative cultures to talk about menstruation (or menopause) with male clinicians.

Death

While talking about impending death is not an easy thing for any person, it is relatively acceptable if the subject is skillfully broached. However, it is not a welcome subject to bring up with patients in many cultures. In Asia, it is expected that the issue will only be discussed with family members, who will then *protect* the patient. However, in its extreme (as in Micronesia), it is taboo even to inquire about death in relation to a person who is already deceased. Clinicians cannot ask whether the parents are still alive or have died, or to ask about the cause of death of grandparents. Clinicians will do best by touching upon the subject indirectly, hinting to the patient, and waiting for the patient to bring it up himself or herself.

The Physical Examination

The physical examination is a required part of a contemporary medical examination. Yet, this is not so in some traditional medical practices. In traditional Chinese medicine, in addition to the oral history, holding the patient's wrist to examine the pulse is the only physical contact that needs to be made by the physician. Historically in China, not even such minimal contact was allowed by (male) physicians in examining the emperor's wife. Instead a string was tied to the emperor's wife's wrist and the physician held the string through a screen to examine the pulse. In other words, direct physical contact was not allowed, or minimally so, even though it was needed for medical diagnosis.

A case example: An elderly Chinese-American man refused to go back to see an internist for a needed follow-up visit. In spite of his family's encouragement, he adamantly refused, only agreeing to see a traditional Chinese medical doctor. He eventually revealed that the Western doctor gave him a *painful* examination at the first visit, and he did not want to go back to see that doctor anymore. He reported that the doctor stuck a finger into his *lower part*. It was not only painful, but it was humiliating. Apparently, the internist, being put off by the patient's poor English, had not effectively explained the purpose of doing a rectal examination, including a prostate check. The patient preferred the methods of traditional Chinese medicine doctors who only take a patient's pulse for the examination.

Most patients understand and accept the intrusion on their personal boundaries that occur during a medical examination, even when they would not accept such bodily contact in any other situation. Sometimes, however, cultural considerations become important not only related to the perception and reaction to the intrusion beyond personal boundaries, but also to the meaning of the parts of the body, including which parts are considered *private* or *erotic*. Furthermore, private or erotic zones may differ among cultural groups and require additional sensitivity and respect to preserve the dignity and comfort of the patient and his or her family. For traditional Japanese women, the back of the neck is not private, but is considered erotic to men, and it may be exposed when women wear traditional clothes (*kimono*), particularly by *geisha*. The chest, especially the breasts, including the upper part of the breasts, however, is considered a very private part of the body and is ordinarily not exposed. Similarly, traditional Muslim women may consider it important to cover their hair and face with a veil, and this may be true even during a physical exam.

In some remote Micronesian islands, adolescent girls and adult women go topless, only wearing grass or cloth skirts around the waist. Yet, for them, it is very important not to expose their body between the navel and the knee. For a clinician to perform a physical examination of a female in this area of the body, it is necessary to have the husband (if married) or mother or older sister (if not yet married) to be present to insure that the clinician will perform the examination professionally without any improper intention.

How a male physician should carry out the physical examination of a female patient is, of course, of special concern in all medical practice. In the United States, professional custom increasingly dictates that a female nurse be present for both the patient's ease as well as for prevention of malpractice suits. In some cultures, it is also expected that the husband will be present when his wife is examined by a male physician. The professional implications of a female physician examining a male patient need to be considered from a cultural perspective as well.

Boundaries of the body differ among people of different cultural groups. It is not the actual body boundary but the sense of self boundary—termed *symbolic skin* by the medical anthropologist, Helman (2000, p. 15). He divides the symbolic skin into several different invisible boundaries—circles of space and distance surrounding the actual bodies. The *intimate distance* can be entered by those who have an intimate physical relationship with the individual; *personal distance* can be entered by those who are not quite as intimate; and *social distance* is the distance at which impersonal business transactions and casual social interactions take place. These different distances vary markedly between people of different cultural groups. For example, for middle-class Americans, close physical contact is allowed between couples or lovers not only in private settings but also in public, while reasonable social distance needs to be maintained among ordinary acquaintances. In contrast, intimate physical contact is avoided in public settings in Japan—even between husband and wife—but close *personal distance* is permitted between colleagues, particularly when they are having a good time after drinking together. Also, close *social distance* is tolerated in a crowded subway or bus even though a certain distance should be kept in ordinary social settings.

Healthcare providers doing physical examinations or treating or caring for the body, are entering (or intruding) into the culturally allowed personal distance. The implications of, and possible psychological reactions toward, this intrusion into the boundaries of the body deserve careful attention and management.

Pelvic Examination

Rarely, but occasionally, a physician (usually a gynecologist) may be asked by parents to perform a pelvic examination on their daughter—not strictly for medical purposes, but for social or cultural reasons: to check her virginity. The following is a case example of such a circumstance.

A Mexican 16-year old girl was brought by her parents to see a gynecologist to verify whether her hymen was still intact and she was still a virgin. According to the parents' culture, virginity is very important and must be saved and protected until the marriage take place. It is desired that the husband have a *sexually intact* bride. The parents were distressed that their teenage daughter was out more often recently and, in spite of the parents' restrictive order, she was coming home late. They tried to force their daughter to tell them what was happening outside, whether she already had a boyfriend or not, but the daughter would not tell them anything and kept denying that anything bad had happened. Offering no options, the parents forced their daughter to go to the doctor to be examined.

The gynecologist felt uncomfortable in this awkward situation. He explained to the parents that it is not his professional task to perform an examination for such a purpose. Even if he performed the examination, he was ethically required to keep the findings confidential, not informing the parents unless the daughter wanted this and agreed to allow it. Furthermore, the doctor took the opportunity to educate the parents that society (and culture) was different in the United States. Youngsters often experience sexual activities early, and concern about virginity prior to marriage was not something to worry about. Providing sexual education and preventing pregnancy or sex-related diseases were the important matters for young people. The parents were very upset at this response from the doctor, and refused to let their daughter see him.

A better outcome might have been achieved if the doctor had found a way to be sensitive to the culture-based needs of the parents while maintaining the proper role as an advocate and confidant for the patient. The doctor could have listened carefully and seriously to the parents, and then offered to see the daughter privately. Informing the daughter about the confidential nature of his evaluation, he could assess the daughter's situation, counsel her as necessary, and examine her if appropriate, with her permission. He could then talk to the parents after explaining to the daughter what he would say, and getting her permission. He could then tell the parents something like "I have good news. Your daughter is healthy. I provided some counseling that I think will be useful for her. She seems to be a wonderful girl, and you should be proud of her." If, as occasionally happens, significant sexually-related problems are found, a recommendation and referral for further counseling can be made.

Diagnostic Tests

While most patients submit to various forms of testing without complaint, occasionally one becomes distressed or even refuses certain tests, such as the claustrophobic patient who refuses an MRI. Cultural factors are sometimes involved in these adverse reactions to diagnostic testing. The following is a case example.

An elderly Asian-American woman insisted on being discharged from the hospital against medical advice. After careful inquiry by the nurse, the patient replied that she did not mind just laying in bed all day, and she could put up with the taste-less food, understanding that she was sick and needed care, but she could not tolerate having her blood drawn every morning. It was not the pain from the needle, but she feared that the loss of blood would prevent recovery and make her sicker. She was certain in her belief that blood was a critical body fluid—the essence of *vitality*. After careful explanations were given to her, a promise to maintain her vitality was made. Her food order was changed so that every morning she could have one *nutritious* egg that would replenish her withdrawn body essence and vitality. She then agreed to stay in the hospital, and agreed to having her blood drawn daily as needed to check her medical condition.

A similar situation may apply to spinal taps when spinal fluid—the essence of the *spirit*—is drawn for testing. In contrast, providing urine, feces, or sputum for testing is extremely unlikely to be a problem, because they are recognized as waste.

To promote or maintain health, many preventative medicine guidelines have been proposed, and various health examinations and tests have been recommended. Yet, people of various backgrounds may not follow such health guidelines faithfully and will not take suggested disease-prevention measures regularly. Ethnic, cultural minority, and socioeconomic factors need to be considered, among others. For instance, in relation to ethnic differences in breast-cancer screening behaviors, Friedman, Webb, Weinberg, Lane, Cooper, and Woodruff (1995) examined asymp-tomatic women 50 years or older who participated in a no cost, worksite breast cancer screening program. The results indicated that African-Americans and Hispanic-Americans were more likely to practice monthly breast self-examination than were Caucasian-Americans. African-Americans were more likely to report cancer-related fears and worries as barriers to having mammography examinations, whereas Caucasian-Americans were more likely to report being too busy, inconven-ience, and procrastination as barriers.

In conclusion, cultural issues permeate the process of clinical assessment. Attention to these issues will increase the likelihood of full patient cooperation and a satisfactory assessment.

References

Carpenter V, Colwell B (1995) Cancer knowledge, self-efficacy, and cancer screening behaviors among Mexican-American women. Journal of Cancer Education 10(4):217–222

Chavez LR, Hubbell FA, McMullin JM, Martinez RG, Mishra SI (1995) Archives of Family Medicine 4(2):145–152

Dancy B (1996) What African-American women know, do, and feel about AIDS: A function of age and education. AIDS Education and Prevention 8(1):26–36

Fernandez ES, South-Paul JE, Matheny SC (2003) Culture, race, and ethnicity issues in health-care. In: Taylor RB (ed) Family Medicine: Principles and Practice. Springer, New York, (pp 17–23

Friedman LC, Webb JA, Weinberg AD, Lane M, Cooper HP, Woodruff A (1995) Breast cancer screen-ing: Racial/ethic differences in behaviors and beliefs. Journal of Cancer Education 10(4):213–216

Hodes RM, Teferedegne B (1996) Traditional beliefs and disease practices of Ethiopian Jews. Israel Journal of Medical Science 32(7):561–567

Hubbell FA, Chavez LR, Mishra SI, Valdez RB (1996) Beliefs about sexual behavior and other predictors of Papanicolaou smear screening among Latinas and Anglo women. Archives of Internal Medicine 156(20):2353–2358

Lee E (1997) Cross-cultural communication: Therapeutic use of interpreters. In: Lee E (ed) Working with Asian Americans: A Guide for Clinicians. Guiford, New York, pp 477–489

Luk S (2006) Overcoming language barriers in psychiatric practice: Culturally-sensitive and effective use of interpreters. In: The Proceedings of the First World Congress of Cultural Psychiatry. S-III-30

Matsumoto D, Pun KK, Nakatani M, Kadowaki D, Weissman M, McCarter L, Fletcher D, Takeuchi S (1995) Cultural differences in attitudes, values, and beliefs about osteoporosis in first and second generation Japanese-American women. Women Health 23:39–56

Morgan C, Park E, Cortes DE (1995) Beliefs, knowledge, and behavior about cancer among urban Hispanic women. In: National Cancer Institute Monographs.(18):57–63

Streltzer J (2004) Culture and consultation-liaison psychiatry. In: Tseng WS, Streltzer J (eds) Clinical Competence in Cultural Psychiatry. American Psychiatric Press, Washington D.C., pp 73–75

Tseng WS (2001) Handbook of Cultural Psychiatry. Academic Press, San Diego, 113

Woollet A, Dosanjh N, Nicolson P, Marshall H, Djhanbakhch O, Hadlow J (1995) The ideas and experiences of pregnancy and childbirth of Asian and non-Asian women in east London. British Journal of Medical Psychology 68(1):65–84

Chapter 4
Healthcare for People of Different Ethnicities

Medical issues that are relatively specific to certain ethnic groups will be discussed in this chapter. For each ethnic group discussed, we will give a brief socio-cultural history, biological variations, frequently encountered medical disorders, common beliefs relating to health and/or illness, folk healing practices, and suggestions for the clinical care of such patients.

It is impossible to exhaustively review all ethnic groups that exist worldwide, so only certain ethnic groups in the United States will be examined here. They are representative of minor or major ethnic groups identified for the purpose of administration and convenience for public data analysis. It needs to be cautioned that, even within an identified particular ethnic group there exist many heterogeneous subgroups, and there are many people with mixed ethnic backgrounds associated with interethnic marriages. Furthermore, there exist wide individual variations within groups, so ethnic stereotypes must be avoided in the evaluation and management of any given individual. However, a general description of some commonly observed health-related behaviors or medically-related phenomena relevant to particular ethnic groups will help provide a basis for understanding their healthcare needs.

African-Americans

Overview

The term *African-American* refers to the descendents of people who were brought to America from Africa during the era of slavery between the 16th and 19th centuries (Black 1996). It also includes recent black immigrants from the African continent (Egypt, Ethiopia, Ghana, Nigeria), the Caribbean (Barbados, Haiti, Tinidad), and Central America (Panama).

The percentage of African-Americans in the United States was 11.9 percent in the year 2000; it is projected to be 14.0 percent in 2020 and 15.4 percent in 2050 (U.S. Bureau of the Census 2001). After the Civil War, when slaves were liberated, many African-Americans migrated from southern rural areas to northern urban areas, although more than half the population has remained in the South. Even though many African-Americans are successful in professional careers and are becoming increasingly affluent, they are relatively poor when considered in aggregate. In 1999, about 22 percent of African-American families had incomes below the poverty line, compared to only 10 percent of all U.S. families at large (U.S. Bureau of the Census 2001). Many African-Americans still live in segregated neighborhoods.

Slavery altered family structure and, indeed, most aspects of life (Black 1996). Although being a single head of household is accepted without associated stigma in African-American families, single parenting and poverty are causal factors in destabilizing the African-American family. Poverty and incarceration are three times higher among black males than among their white counterparts (Glanville 2003, p 43). A growing number of African-American grandparents are functioning in primary parental roles. Many African-American families, especially those with a single head of household, are matrifocal in nature, and the healthcare provider must recognize a woman's often overriding importance in decision-making and disseminating health information.

Biological Variations

Biologically, African-Americans are a very heterogeneous group. They encompass a gene pool of over 100 racial strains (Goddard 1990). Therefore, for instance, skin color among African-Americans can vary from light to very dark. Assessing the skin of most African-American patients requires different clinical skills from those for assessing people with white skin. For example, pallor in dark-skinned African-Americans can be observed by the absence of the underlying red tones that give the brown and black skin its *glow* or *living color*. Lighter-skinned African Americans will appear more yellowish brown, whereas darker-skinned African Americans appear ashen. To assess the skin conditions of inflammation, cyanosis, jaundice, and petechiae may require natural light and the use of different assessment skills (Glanville 2003, pp 44–45).

African-Americans have a tendency toward the overgrowth of connective tissue associated with protection against infection and repair after injury. Keloid formation is one example of this tendency. Lymphoma and systematic lupus erythematosus occur in African-Americans secondary to this overgrowth of connective tissue.

Bone density is another biological variation noted among African-Americans. They have higher bone density than other ethnic groups such as European, Asian, and Hispanic-Americans. Their long bones are longer as well. They experience a lower incidence of osteoporosis (Glanville 2003, p 45).

Medical Disorders

The pathophysiology of hypertension in African-Americans is related to volume expansion, decreased renin, and increased intracellular concentration of sodium and calcium. Genetically, African-Americans are more prone than Caucasian-Americans to retaining sodium. Therefore, a high intake of sodium, extra weight, a sedentary lifestyle, smoking, alcohol, and high stress levels are associated with increased blood pressure, which is a particularly common health problem among African-Americans (Stewart, Johnson & Saunders 2006).

African-Americans suffer from certain genetic-related diseases. Sickle cell anemia is the most common genetic disorder among the African-American population. Glucose-6-phospate dehydrogenase deficiency, which interferes with glucose metabolism, is another example. Hypertension, cancer of the esophagus, stomach cancer, coccidioidomycosis, and lactose intolerance are some of the medical problems more often seen in African-American patients.

AIDS contributes more to lowering the life expectancy of African-Americans than it does to European-Americans. According to the Center for Disease Control, a larger percentage of African-Americans are infected with HIV and are dying from AIDS than ny other ethnic groups in the United States (Glanville 2003, p 46).

High-risk behaviors among African-Americans can be inferred from the high incidence of HIV/AIDS and other sexually transmitted diseases, teenage pregnancy, violence, unintentional injuries, smoking, alcoholism, drug abuse, sedentary lifestyle, and delayz in seeking healthcare.

Health Beliefs and Practice

Many African-Americans, particularly those of low-income, have been described as holding beliefs about illness that can be separated into two categories (Snow 1983). *Natural illness* occurs as a result of God's will, or when a person comes into unhealthy contact with the force of nature, such as exposure to cold or impurities in the air, food, or water. A cure for natural illness includes an antidote or other logical protective actions. *Unnatural illness*, on the other hand, is considered the result of evil influence that alters God's intended plan. Treatment or cures for unnatural illness can be found in religion, magic, amulets, and herbs. African-Americans have long used prayer and religiosity to cope with and treat health concerns (Welch 2003, pp 40). Although praying and *letting God take care of things* is a major emotional support for many African-Americans (especially among elderly women), it can often lead to delays in seeking professional healthcare.

Some Issues Relating to Clinical Care

Many African-Americans perceive white (Caucasian-Americans) healthcare professionals as outsiders, and they may resent them for telling them what their problems are or telling them how to solve them (Underwood 1994). African-Americans may be suspicious and cautious of healthcare practitioners they have not heard of or do not know. It is important to initially focus on developing a trusting relationship.

A recent study of elderly African-Americans attempted to determine what these patients considered culturally competent care. Most thought that it was important for physicians to know something about African-American culture, but only in the context of medical or healthcare issues. To be culturally competent, the ethnicity or sex of the doctor was less important than the ability to provide appropriate diagnosis and treatment while communicating clearly and showing respect (Johnson, Slusar, Chaatre & Johnsen 2006).

Because African-Americans are more likely to have lower socioeconomic status, they more often experience economic barriers to healthcare services. For example, the diet prescribed by the American Diabetic Association is geared for Caucasian (or European)-Americans without consideration for the dietary habits of other ethnic groups, including African-Americans (Glanville 2003, p 50). Such a diet is likely to be more expensive, and thus both economic and cultural barriers prevent patients from adhering to the recommended diet.

Most clinical drug trials primarily use Caucasian-American subjects. Responses from other ethnic groups—regarding the efficacy of the drugs and side effects— may not be well-studied. Of the drugs that have been studied across ethnic groups, some are metabolized differently by African-Americans as a group, including alcohol, antihypertensives, beta blockers, psychotropic drugs, and caffeine.

Like many ethnic groups, African-Americans utilize folk medicine. For them, folk practitioners can be spiritual leaders, grandparents, elders of the community, voodoo doctors, or priests. African-Americans may use home remedies to maintain their health and treat specific health conditions.

Native American Groups

Overview

The term *Native-American* refers broadly to American Indians, Alaska natives, native Hawaiians, and those who were pre-Columbian inhabitants of North America. These groups are enormously diverse. They share a common historical path, however, in that they suffered from massive decimation of their people, loss of ancestral lands, and destruction of their languages, cultures, and religions (Norton & Manson 1996). The loss of more than 90 percent of their population was due to wars, genocide, and disease (such as smallpox and influenza) from contact with Europeans (Trimble, Fleming, Beauvais & Jumper-Thurman 1996). Based on the information available, the discussion herein will focus mainly on American Indians, even though the other Native Americans will be touched upon occasionally.

At present, American Indians and Native Alaskans comprised slightly less than 1 percent of the American population (U.S. Census Bureau 1995). However, there are more than 250 federally recognized American Indian tribes and 225 native Alaskan villages. Most American Indians live in the Western states—including California, Arizona, New Mexico, South Dakota, Alaska, and Montana—with 42 percent residing in rural areas compared to 23 percent of whites (Department of Health and Human Services 2001). Over half of American Indians live in urban areas, and those on reservations may spend time away seeking education, jobs, and other opportunities. Therefore, major cities have a substantial American Indian population (Sutton & Nose 1996).

Following the devastation of these once-thriving Indian nations, the social environments of native people have remained plagued by economic disadvantage. Many American Indians and Alaskan natives are unemployed or hold low-paying jobs (Department of Health and Human Services 2001). About 26 percent of American Indians and Alaskan natives live in poverty, as compared to 13 percent for the United States as a whole, and 8 percent for Caucasian (European)-Americans (U.S. Census Bureau 1999).

Common Concepts and Beliefs Relating to Health and Illness

Traditionally, American Indians have a world view that there is no relevant difference between the natural and the supernatural. These concepts are mixed, and work together. There is a fundamental equality between human beings and their environment. There is a personalized and dynamic interaction between humans, spirits, and power. Ritual is used to harness and manipulate power. Therefore, medicine, religion, and magic may be closely related in the mind of American Indian (Daley & Daley 2003, pp 100–106). In general, wellness means harmony of body, mind, and spirit, and unwellness means disharmony among them. However, the concept of physical illness varies with individual adherence to traditional medicine or Western biomedicine. Navajo traditions may relate physical illness to violations of social proscriptive behaviors (Kramer 1996, p 20).

Common Medical Disorders

Heart disease, liver cirrhosis, and diabetes mellitus are some of the chronic medical disorders particularly prevalent in the Native American population. The leading causes of death for American Indians are cardiovascular diseases, malignant neoplasms, accidents and cirrhosis (associated with drinking), diabetes, cerebrovascular diseases, pneumonia and influenza, and suicide. Alcoholism or substance abuse is relatively high among Native Americans—particularly among young people. Alcohol and substance abuse are associated with high rates of violence and accidents.

Issues Related to Healthcare

American Indians suffer some of the worst health in the nation. Access to healthcare is more difficult for many because of geographic isolation in villages and communities within large reservation areas. These areas may have poor transportation, lack of efficient communication systems, and lack of environmental hygiene associated with the absence of running water and sewage disposal systems. To reach a health clinic, they may need to travel for long distances on dirty roads. Regular follow-up may be impossible due to such conditions (Fernandez, South-Paul & Matheny 2003, p 19). The situation is similar for other Native Americans, including the Pacific Islanders.

Language and Communication

American Indians consider speaking too quickly and too loudly as signs of disrespect. For some groups, it is taboo to speak the name of a deceased individual. It is believed that speaking the name alerts the person's spirit, which can bring misfortune and harm. One way to avoid this taboo is to use kinship terminology, such as *maternal grandmother*. Another common taboo is against speaking too much about an illness, which is believed to make that illness worse (Daley & Daley 2003, pp 119–120).

Pain

American Indians commonly hold the view that complaining of pain is a sign of weakness. Therefore, they will avoid complaining of pain directly and explicitly, and refer to pain indirectly in general terms, such as: "I don't feel so good," or "Something doesn't feel right." If a patient reports being *uncomfortable* and gets no pain relief, the patient is unlikely to repeat the request for assistance. The patient may complain of pain to trusted family members or visitors with the hope that they will relay the message to a healthcare worker (Kramer 1996, p 15).

Attitude Toward Western Medicine

Relationships between American Indians and whites have often been poor. This is partly based on the historical path, and it is partly due to white ethnocentrism. For most American Indians, medicine and religion are tightly interwoven. Many believe that the cause of illness is rooted in the spirit world, and that the spirit world must likewise be involved in its cure. In addition to the gap between the basic orientation of native medicine and Western medicine, many American Indians consider biomedicine to be an extension of prior colonialism. Extra effort to work through this barrier may be necessary when healthcare workers of European American background provide healthcare for these native peoples.

Muslims and Arab Americans

Overview

The term *Muslim* refers to people who practice the Islam religion, while *Arab* refers to people whose ancestors come from a specific geographic region. Therefore, Arabic people are not necessarily Muslims, and Muslims are not necessarily Arabs. Many Muslims live outside of Arab countries, such as in Indonesia, Pakistan, India, Malaysia, and many African countries. In the United States, Muslims represent many ethnicities, including most Arab-Americans. For the sake of convenience, therefore, Muslims and Arab-Americans will be grouped together for discussion here because they share the common characteristics of the Islamic faith (Hammound & Siblani 2003, pp 161–167). The situation for people in the homeland of Arab societies will be quoted because it often reflects the root of behavior for many Arab Americans.

Islam is one of the three major monotheistic religions in the world. It is classified as a religion, but it is actually a way of life—affecting everything from personal hygiene to patterns of socialization. Muslims structure their lives based on five pillars of Islam. These are: proclamation of one's belief in the one and only God and in Mohammed's status as the last messenger of God; the obligatory performance of prayer five times every day following certain guidelines on form, content, and time; payment of a religious tax to care for the needy in the community and partly to fulfill other objectives for the collective good; observation of the month of Ramadan and the associated fasting; and the pilgrimage to Mecca at least once in a lifetime (Hammoud & Siblani 2003, pp 169–171).

Arabic Muslim families are characterized by a patrilineal tradition, with strong emphasis on hierarchy based on age and gender. Women are subordinate to men, and young people to older people. Within the family, the man is the head and his influence is overt. In public, a wife's interactions with her husband are formal and respectful. However, behind the scenes, she typically wields tremendous influence, particularly in matters pertaining to the home and children (Kulwicki 2003, p 93).

Common Concepts, Beliefs, and Attitudes Relating to Health

For Arabs, health is viewed as a gift of God manifested by being able to eat well, having a good mood without pain or stress, and having the strength to meet social obligations. Being overweight is associated with health and strength (Meleis 1996, P 35). Physical illness is seen by folk people to be caused by an *evil eye*, bad luck, sudden fears, stress in family, loss of person or objects, germs, wind and draft, and an imbalance in hot, dry, cold, and moist. Among children, deprivations are considered as the cause of illness (Meleis 1996, p 34).

Traditional Islamic medicine is based on the theory of four humors—black bile, blood, phlegm, and yellow bile—and the primary attributes of dryness, heat, cold, and moisture. Illness is viewed as an imbalance between them. Therapy involves treating with the disease's opposite. For example, a cold remedy is used for hot disease (Kulwicki 2003).

Good health is seen as the ability to fulfill one's roles. Arabs are expected to express and acknowledge their ailments when they are ill. Muslims often mention that the Prophet urged physicians to perform research and the ill to seek treatment because "Allah has not created a disease without providing care for it," except for the problem of old age. However, despite this belief that one should care for health and seek treatment when ill, Arab women are often reluctant to seek care. Because of the cultural emphasis placed on modesty, some women are very reluctant to disrobe for an examination.

Cultural Considerations Relating to Some Medical Practices

In Arab societies, males and females have distinct roles, and there is frequent segregation between genders. Unrelated males and females are not accustomed to interacting. Shyness in women is appreciated, and Muslim men may ignore women out of politeness. Healthcare settings, clinics, and sometimes waiting rooms are segregated by sex. Male nurses never care for female patients. Some families object to female family members being examined by male physicians. Given this background, many Arab-Americans may find interacting with a healthcare professional of the opposite sex quite embarrassing and stressful. Discomfort may be expressed by refusal to discuss personal information and by a reluctance to disrobe for physical exams and hygienic procedures (Kulwicki 2003).

When language is an issue, it is best to use same-sex interpreters whenever possible. If a family member is used for translation of sensitive topics related to marital problems, sex, reproduction, or highly sensitive disease such as cancer, HIV/AIDS, tuberculosis, or venereal disease, a relative of the same sex is preferable. One should be aware that family members serving as interpreters may edit communications to the patient, thinking they are protecting the patient. (Meleis 1996, p 25).

Although most American healthcare professionals consider full disclosure an ethical obligation, most Arabic people do not believe that it is necessary for a patient to know how serious a diagnosis is or the full details of a surgical procedure. In fact, communicating a grave diagnosis is often viewed as cruel and tactless because it deprives the patient of hope. Similarly, preoperative instructions and information are thought to cause needless anxiety (Kulwicki 2003).

Arabic people expect physicians to have the expertise to select proper treatment. Apart from the educated, most patients are not interested in actively participating in decision-making for their medical treatment (Abu Gharbeih 1993). The patient's role is to cooperate. The authority of physicians is seldom challenged or questioned. When treatment is successful, the physician's skill is recognized. Adverse outcomes are attributed to God's will unless there is evidence of blatant malpractice.

Arabs and Arab-Americans are in general very expressive about pain, particularly in the presence of family members with whom they feel comfortable. Pain is feared and causes panic when it occurs. They expect to avoid pain at all cost. For medical treatment, they believe that injection is more effective than pills. However, some may perceive intravenous fluids as an indication of a situation's severity. Alcohol-containing liquid medications may be avoided by Muslims, based on their religious beliefs about not consuming alcohol.

Although blood transfusions and organ transplants are widely accepted, organ donation is a controversial issue among Arabs and Arab-Americans. Practices of organ donation may vary among Arab Muslims and non-Muslims based on their religious beliefs about death and dying, reincarnation, or their personal feelings about helping others by donating their organs to others or for scientific purpose. Physicians should be sensitive to personal, family, or religious practices toward organ donation among Arab-Americans and should not make any assumptions about organ donation without carefully consulting family members (Kulwicki 2003, p 102).

Male circumcision is expected. Some prefer it when a son is about six years old, while others prefer it being done on newborns in the hospital before discharge. Female circumcision is never discussed at birth. If the subject comes up, it usually arises when a daughter is school age or an adolescent. Female circumcision is not based on religious beliefs, but is passed on culturally. Contemporary Arab-Americans usually do not attempt to have their young daughters circumcised. Some females, however, may have been circumcised in their home country before coming to the United States (Meleis 1996, pp 30–31).

Regarding death, Arabs do not openly anticipate or grieve before death occurs. The sensitive physician will do well to inform the head of a family privately of an impending death, allowing him to decide how to inform the rest of family. Deciding whether or not to resuscitate a patient at the terminal stage is often difficult. The family may lose trust in the healthcare system if the option of "Do Not Resuscitate (DNR)" is offered to them (Meleis 1996, p 31). Instead, the physician should clearly recommend the best course of action based on the clinical situation.

Asian-American Groups

Overview

Asian-Americans refer broadly to people originally from China, Japan, Korea, or Southeast Asia—such as the Philippines, Vietnam, Laos, Cambodia, Thailand, and India. Sometimes Pacific Islanders from Micronesia (Guam), Hawaii, and Samoa are included in this group for statistical purposes. Outsiders refer to all of these people as *Asian* because they have a superficially similar appearance, but actually they belong to diverse groups with different languages and cultures, histories of migration, and levels of acculturation to the host society (Kitano & Maki 1996).

Asian people generally value family, and emphasize group orientation, collectivism, and interdependence among members of task-oriented groups. Cooperation, compromising, and keeping harmony are valued. The assumption of a middle position is encouraged in dealing with situations—avoiding extremes. For interpersonal relations, hierarchy and respect for elders is emphasized.

Common Concepts and Beliefs Relating to Health

The folk medicine concepts shared by many Asian-Americans are more or less rooted in Chinese traditional medicine that has had a wide impact in Asia for several centuries. There are basic concepts involved in Chinese traditional medicine.

The Concept of Yin and Yang

The world is seen as composed of two basic forces—*yin* and *yang*—not only for the environment, but also for the human being. As an extension of this worldview, traditional medicine perceives a balance between *yin* and *yang* as necessary for well-being, with an imbalance between them leading to sickness.

The Theory of Five Elements

In addition to the concept of *yin* and *yang*, traditional Chinese medicine also holds the theory of five elements—water, wood, fire, earth, and metal. The universe is composed of these basic elements. The five elements correspond to five visceral organs—kidney, heart, liver, spleen, and lung. These, in turn, correspond to five emotions—fear, joy, anger, worry, and sorrow. There is a circular relationship and paired antagonisms among the five elements.

Organ-rooted dysfunction

Traditionally, everything occurring in the body and mind was interpreted as an expression of the visceral organs. Many excessive emotional and somatic symptoms were interpreted as the result of dysfunction in the visceral organs. The folk idioms of *empty heart, elevated liver fire, explosion of spleen force*, and *insufficient kidney* are used in daily life among laymen to express various emotional problems or somatic discomforts. Conceptually, mind and body are not separated in Asia as they are in Western dualism. Presenting health complaints may reflect this mind-body unity.

Etiology of Illness

Causal factors producing sickness are conceptually placed into three basic categories—namely external, internal, and others. External causes refer to any illness arising from injury or forces of nature (such as exceptionally windy conditions, high humidity, and excessive heat or cold). Internal causes refer to factors arising from inside a person (improper emotional experiences). Others include those causes not explained by external and internal causes. Physical disorders affect the emotions and, at the same time, problematic emotional experiences result in illness.

The Concept of Vital Energy

A vital force, called *jing* (essence of energy) in Chinese, or *genki* (vital air) in Japanese, exists in the body and regulates the life of the organism. When a person is full of vital energy, he functions efficiently both mentally and physically. Without sufficient vital energy, however, illness and even death may occur.

Medical Disorders More Common in Asians

Liver, esophagus, and stomach cancer are more prevalent among Asian-Americans. Hepatitis B is relatively high among new immigrants from South Asia. Lactose intolerance is a medical problem for many. Pulmonary tuberculosis is more prevalent in Asian-Americans, especially first generation immigrants. The overall rate for Asian-Americans is 25.5 per 100,000 population, which is greater than that for other minorities. Their numbers are 10.8 for African-Americans, 9.4 for Hispanic-Americans, and 8.2 for American Indians. The rate for Caucasians is 1.3 per 100,000 (Center for Disease Control and Prevention 2006).

Cultural Considerations in Certain Medical Issues

Seeking Care

Asians may not feel a particular obligation to stay with one family doctor. They may be comfortable shopping around and changing physicians. They may see several physicians simultaneously, including traditional practitioners.

Using Traditional Medicine

Chinese traditional medicine has a very long history and is still commonly used even by educated patients. In addition to Western medication, Asian patients may simultaneously use herb medicine, take tonics, and receive acupuncture. Traditional elderly Japanese may receive *okiu* (moxibustion- burning the skin with herbs) as a special remedy from traditional healers.

Pharmacological Considerations

Asian patients, as a group, metabolize some medications at a different rate than Caucasians, but there is great individual variation. Clinical experience dictates that, in general, Asian patients often need only about half the dose typical for Caucasian patients to achieve the same therapeutic effects. The Asian patient may suffer from more severe side effects at doses suggested for Caucasian patients.

Informing the Patient about a Terminal Prognosis

In general, Asian families prefer the physician not to directly inform the patient of a terminal prognosis, out of concern that the *weak* patient may not be able to deal with the *bad* news. This tendency of concealing the prognosis from patients is gradually changing. A similar trend occurred in the United States about 50 years ago (Oken 1961).

Caucasian-American Groups

Overview

The term Caucasian has several meanings and interesting historical roots. In the United States, the term has been used to refer to the majority racial category. The term is gradually being replaced by *white* or *European-American*. The terms *Caucasian-American* and *European-American* are interchangeably used here (Maretzki and McDermott, 1980). These groups of people in the United States are descendents of (Western) European nationals (mainly British, French, German, Greek, and Italian, but not Spain or Portugal). Because of their fair skin, they are called *white* in contrast to other nonwhite ethnic groups. Due to historical reasons and administrative custom, descendents of Spain or those with Latin background are identified as Hispanic-Americans and discussed separately.

European-Americans are the major and dominant group in the United States. There are 53 categories of European-Americans, of which the largest are German-Americans (58 million), those of English ancestry (British, English, Welsh, and Scottish—41 million), and Irish Americans (39 million) (Giordano & McGoldrick

1996, p 427). Most families of European-American groups have been in the United States for three generations or more. An increasing number have intermarried with other European ethnic groups, and often are unaware of and uninterested in their mixed European heritage—thinking of themselves simply as *Americans*.

Even though European-Americans are composed of many ethnic groups, they, as a whole, are regarded mainly as *white* by nonwhite people, or as *Westerners* by *Easterners*, and are considered to have some common cultural traits. In general, they—as the mainstream of the country (United States, and also Canada)—have been described as being individually oriented (in contrast to situation or collectively oriented); present- or future-oriented (rather than past-oriented); oriented to actively and aggressively solving problems (rather than passively or submissively tolerating or accepting them); oriented to challenges and trying to conquer in their relationships with nature (rather than trying to comply or be in harmony with nature).

Looking more closely, however, Caucasian-Americans are composed of different ethnic groups that have distinguishable historical heritage and cultural backgrounds. A few of the subgroups will be selected here for brief discussion with particular concern relevant to healthcare issues.

Irish-Americans

Irish-Americans have ancestors from Ireland. The great majority identify as Catholic (McGoldrick 1982). The Irish immigrated to America in large numbers for almost three centuries beginning in the 1600s. The threat of famine, religious persecution (from Protestants), and deplorable economic conditions were primary reasons for early immigration. Immigration to the United States from Ireland was so substantial that there are now more Irish-Americans than there are Irish still living in Ireland. Most Irish immigrants settled in urban industrial areas in the northeastern United States along the Atlantic coast. The history of the Irish in America has not always been harmonious—because they were a religious minority and suffered economic discrimination (from other more affluent European-American groups). Initial experiences of bigotry and prejudice formed the Irish-Americans' values of education, a strong work ethic, and the importance of children. They have made significant contributions in politics, the labor movement, the Catholic Church, the arts, and service to their country (Wilson 2003, pp 194–195).

From a cultural point of view, Church rules were paramount. Suffering (which was to be handled alone) was a punishment for sins, drinking was an important part of social engagements, and complaining about problems was *bad form*. Being self-controlled, strong, and psychologically tough was highly valued. Sex was viewed as dangerous and not to be discussed. As a consequence of sexual repression, they also avoided tenderness, affection, and intimacy between husband and wife (McGoldrick 1982, p 314). Within a family, fathers traditionally were shadowy or absent figures, and husbands dealt with wives primarily by avoidance. In the final analysis, women were expected to take care of things.

The Irish have a reputation for heavy drinking of alcohol and being prone to alcoholism. Numerous theories have been put forth about this. Stevers (1976) commented that the Irish drank heavily in America because they were expected to be heavy drinkers. Family characteristics, social and economic conditions, strong, manipulative Irish mothers, and other psychological issues have been invoked as contributing factors to alcoholism in Irish men.

The Irish are thought to have a fatalistic outlook (external locus of control) that may influence health-seeking behaviors. Many Irish people use denial as a way of coping with physical and psychological problems. A study comparing Irish- and Italian-Americans' perceptions of symptoms of illness suggested that the Irish view of life is illustrated in the belief that: "Life was black and long suffering and the less said about it the better" (Zola 1983).

Many Irish understate their symptoms when they are ill. For some, illness behavior is viewed as doing little to relieve suffering and perpetuates a self-fulfilling prophecy of fatalism. Illness or injury may be linked to guilt and considered to be the result of having done something morally wrong. Restraint is a behavioral norm in the Irish culture—temptation is ever-present and must be guarded against (Zola 1983).

Irish folk medicine practices include traditional remedies that have been passed down through generations and are considered effective in health promotion. These include eating a balanced diet, getting a good night's sleep, exercising, dressing warmly, and not going out in the cold air with wet hair. Other folk practices include wearing religious medals to prevent illness, using cough syrup made from honey and whiskey, taking honey and lemon for a sore throat, drinking hot tea with whiskey for a cold, and putting a damp cloth to the forehead for a headache (Wilson 2003, p 202).

Italian Americans

The early Italians who came to America between the late 18th and 19th centuries were scattered throughout North America, with large concentrations in the Northeast and the lower Mississippi Valley. Early Italian immigrants, mainly from northern Italy, came from an agricultural background and differed in several respects from later immigrants who, mainly from southern Italy, began arriving at the close of the 19th century. Many of the later immigrants were political refugees who had a variety of skills and occupations, such as tradesmen, artists, musicians, and teachers (Hillman 2003, pp 205–206).

From a cultural perspective, Italians considered nothing more important than the family. Eating was a symbol of nurturing and family connectedness and a particular source of enjoyment. At home, roles were separate and defined—men (who were always dominant) protected and women nurtured. Personal connections were the way to get things done. The willingness to share thoughts and feelings among family members is a major distinguishing characteristic of the Italian family. While nonverbal methods of communication are common to all societies, Italians use elaborate, refined, and stylized gestures that are practically an art form.

People of Italian ancestry have some notable genetic diseases, such as familial Mediterranean fever, Mediterranean-type glucose-6-phosphate dehydrogenase deficiency (G-6-PD), and thalassemia (Hillman 2003, p 210). Italian-Americans have a high incidence of hypertension and coronary artery disease. Italian-Americans have significantly higher risks of nasopharyngeal, stomach, liver, and gallbladder tumors (Bernstein, Flannery & Reynolds 1993). Italian-Americans are also at increased risk for multiple sclerosis.

First-generation immigrants are likely to retain traditional health-related beliefs from their area of Italy. Illness, therefore, may be attributed to wind currents that carry disease, contamination, heredity, supernatural or human causes, and psychosomatic interactions. Traditional Italian-Americans believe that people who have disabilities should be cared for at home by the family. Thus, very few individuals are placed in long-term care facilities. For many Italians, the role of being sick is not entered into without personal feelings of guilt—thus, individuals may keep sickness a secret from their family and friends and are not inclined to describe the details because they blame themselves for the health problem. Families may be ashamed to let neighbors know of health-related problems that may impair the social status of a family member.

Earlier Italian immigrants looked questionably on book-trained physicians, and had little trust in American healthcare physicians. With all the folk remedies for cure within easy reach, Italians did not eagerly accept physicians. They considered it rather foolish to pay money just to learn something unpleasant (Hillman 2003, pp 214–216).

Jewish-Americans

The term *Jewish* refers to both a people and a religion—it is not a race. Judaism is both a religion and a culture. Migration of Jews from Europe began to increase in the mid-1800s, often because of the fear of religious persecution. The greatest influx of immigrants occurred between 1880 and 1920. Many of these immigrants came from Russia and Eastern Europe after a wave of anti-Jewish riots and murders, and anti-Jewish decrees (Glazer 1957). Those who migrated from Russia and Eastern Europe are referred as Ashkenazi Jews, in contrast to Sephardic Jews who are originally from Spain, Portugal, North Africa, and South and Central America.

In Jewish culture, children are encouraged to discuss and express their opinions on family problems. They learn that talking about problems is the best way to solve them. Jewish humor is highly valued and has achieved much notoriety. Jewish stereotypes are often the object of such humor, such as the guilt-producing Jewish mother. Success is more highly valued than anything else, and suffering is more easily borne when expressed and shared. A person will get attention when he or she is sick. In the past, Jews rarely married non-Jews, even if they were not religious. In America, this has changed in contemporary generations. For male infants, circumcision (which is both a medical procedure and a religious rite) is still performed. The procedure and the ceremony are performed on the eighth day of life by a person (called a *mohel*) trained in the procedure and the religious ceremony. It is possible to have the procedure done by a physician with a rabbi present to say the blessings (Selekman 2003, p 242).

From the perspective of health and illness, there is a greater incidence of some genetic disorders among individuals of Jewish descent—especially those who are Ashkenazi. Most of these disorders are autosomal recessive, meaning that both parents must carry the affected gene to produce an affected offspring. These disorders include Tay-Sachs disease, Gaucher's disease, Canavan's disease, familial dysautonomia, torsion dystonia, Niemann-Pick disease, Bloom syndrome, Fanconi's anemia, and mucolipidosis IV (National Foundation for Jewish Genetic Disease 2001). Despite the obvious need, a study of genetic counseling services for orthodox Jewish community members revealed that cultural differences and poor communication impeded the ability of the orthodox Jewish community to utilize genetic services. The counselors were apprehensive about serving this community, and were unaware of cultural traditions and norms (Mittman, Bowie & Maman 2007).

Concerning healthcare-related spiritual beliefs, one of the Ten Commandments is to remember the Sabbath day and keep it holy. The Sabbath begins 18 minutes before sunset Friday and ends 42 minutes after sunset on Saturday. If an orthodox patient's condition is not life-threatening, medical and surgical procedures should not be performed on the Sabbath or holy days. However, matters involving human life take precedence. In ultra-orthodox denominations of Judaism, taking medication on the Sabbath—the day of rest—that is not necessary to preserve life may be viewed as *work*. That is an action performed with the intention of bringing about a change in existing conditions, and is not acceptable. Patients need to be taught about the potential life-threatening consequences of their condition, as well as the exceptions to Jewish law that permit them to take their medication (Selekman 2003, p 246).

For Jewish people, the verbalization of pain is acceptable and common. Individuals want to know the reason for the pain, which they often consider just as important as obtaining relief from pain. The role of being sick for Jews is highly individualized and may vary among individuals according to the severity of symptoms. The family is central to Jewish life; therefore, family members share the emphasis on maintaining health and assisting with individual responsibilities during times of illness (Selekman 2003, p 246–247). Many Jews have become physicians, psychiatrists, psychoanalysts, and psychologists. In addition, many of their clients are Jewish. Physicians are held in high regard. While physicians must do everything in their power to prolong life, Jewish tradition prohibits them from initiating measures that prolong the act of dying. Once standard therapy has failed, the physician's role changes from that of curer to that of caregiver (Rosner 1993).

The Amish

The Amish are one of the unique subcultural groups found among Caucasian-Americans. In Europe, the Amish emerged after 1693 as a variant of one stream of the Anabaptist movement that originated in Switzerland in 1525 and spread to neighboring German-speaking lands. The Amish name is derived from the surname of Jacob Ammann, who led the Amish division from the Anabaptists in 1693. The Amish embraced, among other Anabaptist tenets of faith, the baptism of adult believers as an outward sign of membership in a voluntary community with an inner commitment to live peacefully with all. Because of their restricted style of dress, activities, and overall life, they appear to others as if they come from another place and a previous time. Amish are *different* by intention and by conviction. They understand their biblical mandate to be living a life separated from a world they see as unregenerate or sinful (Wenger & Wenger 2003, pp 54–55).

Throughout the three centuries of Amish history in North America, the principal and preferred occupations for the Amish have been agricultural work and farm-related enterprises. For the Amish, the kinship network includes consanguine relatives consisting of the parental unit and the households of married children and their offspring. Individuals are identified by their family affiliation. Fondness and love for family members is held deeply, but privately. The expression of joy and suffering is not entirely subdued by stoic silence, but they are not outwardly demonstrative or exuberant.

The Amish do not send their children for higher learning or to pursue professional training. Healthcare professionals, by definition, are outsiders who mediate information on health promotion, make diagnoses, and propose therapies across cultural boundaries. To the extent that they do so with sensitivity and respect for Amish cultural ways, they are respected and valued as an important resource by the Amish (Wenger & Wenger 2003, pp 55). Most Amish consult within their community to learn about physicians, dentists, and nurses with whom they can develop trusting relationships.

The Amish are essentially a closed population, and they marry outsiders very rarely. Although inbreeding is more prevalent in Amish communities, this does not inevitably result in hereditary defects (Hostetler 1993). Nevertheless, several hereditary diseases have been identified among the Amish. They are recessive diseases, including dwarfism, cartilage hair hypoplasia, pyruvate kinase anemia, and hemophilia B.

Amish are traditionally agrarian and prefer a lifestyle that provides intergenerational and community support systems to promote health and to minimize the prevalence of high-risk behaviors. Amish believe that the body is the temple of God and that human beings are the stewards of their bodies. Medicine and healthcare should always be used with the understanding that it is God who heals. Nothing in the Amish understanding of the Bible forbids them from using preventive or curative medical services. The Amish are unlikely to display pain and physical discomfort. The healthcare provider may need to remind the Amish patient that medication is available for pain relief if they choose to accept it. For the Amish, community means inclusion of people who are chronically ill. Amish culture approaches those who need care as a community responsibility.

Hispanic-American Groups

Overview

Hispanic and *Latino* are terms used to refer to Cubans, Chicanos, Mexicans, Puerto Ricans, Argentinians, Colombians, Dominicans, Brazilians, Guatemalans, Costa Ricans, Nicaraguans, Salvadorians, and all the other Spanish-speaking nationalities from South America, Central America, and the Caribbean. Their basic similarities are (except for Brazilians, who speak Portuguese) that most of them speak Spanish, use Spanish surnames, are mostly Roman Catholic, and have common values and beliefs rooted in a history of conquest and colonization. Associated with Latin-American history, Latinos are the descendants of both the oppressors and the oppressed (Garcia-Preto 1996, pp 141–142).

In the United States, they are officially categorized as *Hispanic* by the U.S. Census, while some of them regard the term as an English word without gender, and prefer the terms Latino and Latina. The term Latino is used with the implication that a person is from a Latin American country (e.g., from Cuba). Mexican-Americans tend to prefer the term Latino, because it does not signify a conquering Spain. Some descendants of early Mexican and Spanish settlers, particularly those in New Mexico and Colorado, refer to themselves as *Hispanos*.

Presently in the United States, Mexicans, Puerto Ricans, and Cubans continue to be the three largest Latino groups. There has, however, been an increase in the number of Dominicans, Central Americans, and some South American groups—especially Brazilians. It is projected that Hispanic-Americans will become the largest nonEuropean-American ethnic group in the United States by the year 2020.

Hispanics are highly concentrated in the southwest United States. Their economic status differs to some extent among the three main subgroups, paralleling their educational status. Cuban-Americans are more affluent than Puerto Ricans and Mexican-Americans. The percentage of people below the poverty line is 31 percent for Puerto Ricans, 27 percent for Mexicans, and 14 percent for Cubans (U.S. Census Bureau 2001). Among foreign-born farm workers, the average educational level is only seven years, and little English is spoken. Thus, communication about healthcare issues can be challenging.

Common Concepts and Beliefs Relating to Health

Latinos generally believe that health is controlled by environment, by fate (*distino*), and by the will of God (*las manos de Dios*) (Paula, Lagana & Gonzalez-Ramirez 1996). Many believe that self-care, as advocated in contemporary Western medicine, can adversely affect recovery (by adding this burden on the patient and depleting the energy needed for recovery) and can undermine the care that should be provided by the family. Therefore, hospital restrictions related to visiting or caregiving activities by family are in direct opposition to traditional practices relating to health and can impede the caregiving role of family.

Medical Disorders Common in Hispanics

In the United States, Hispanics are at increased risk for diabetes, hypertension, tuberculosis, HIV infection, alcoholism, cirrhosis, specific cancers, and drinking-related violent deaths. Poverty and lack of health insurance are the greatest impediments to healthcare. One-third to one-fifth of various Hispanic populations in the United States are uninsured for medical expenses, compared with one-tenth of nonHispanic whites (Fernandez, South-Paul & Matheny 2003, P 19).

Mexican-American adults, in contrast to whites, are more likely to be overweight, physically inactive, diabetic, and to have higher levels of hypertension (Afghani, Abbott, Wiswell, Jaque, Gleckner, Schroeder & Johnson 2004). Central adiposity is an important predictor of resting blood pressure in Hispanic women.

In relation to dietary patterns and cardiovascular risk factors, Hispanic adults living in Southwest Detroit were shown to use higher fat salad dressing; eat fried foods, sweets, and high fat snacks; consume greater than the desired amounts of regular cheese; drink whole milk; and eat few fruits and vegetables (Artinian, Schim, Vander, Wal & Nies 2004). In addition, the lack of physical activity, obesity, and exposure to second-hand smoke were the most prevalent cardiovascular risk factors.

Breast cancer is the most commonly diagnosed cancer and the most common cause of cancer mortality of Latino women (Fitzgibon, Gapsture & Knight 2004). Delay in seeking examination and treatment may contribute to these results.

Healthcare Issues

Health Beliefs

Injuries and illnesses may be believed to be due to severe stress, spiritual causes, or conditions such as imbalances of hot and cold. Self-care and alternative healthcare practices may interfere with treatment compliance or outcomes. In many Latin American countries, oral and injectable medications can be purchased without a prescription, which encourages self-care. Alternative healers, such as general healers (*curanderos*), bone-setters (*sobadores*), and witches (*brujos*), may be involved in the care of Latino patients. Alternative and self-care practices should be considered when treating these patients (Poon, Gray, Franco, Cerruti, Schreck & Delgado 2003).

Communication and Relationshisp with Healthcare Providers

Poon, Gray, Franco, Cerruti, Schreck, and Delgado (2003) recommend several factors in maximizing effective communication and culturally competent care. These include showing a genuine interest in the patient and the patient's group, which may include researching the group's background, listening to individual views about healthcare and their difficulties obtaining it, facilitating communication through appropriate interpreters when necessary, and identifying and addressing barriers to healthcare.

Nonverbal communication is strongly influenced by the concept of respect (*respeto*), and therefore direct eye contact is frequently avoided with authority figures such as healthcare providers. Silence sometimes shows lack of agreement with the proposed plan of care. Hispanics tend to be comfortable disagreeing verbally and directly with authority figures, such as doctors. Touch by strangers is generally unappreciated and can be very stressful or perceived as disrespectful. However, physical contact for clinical examination or therapy is performed as an integral part of traditional healing (Paula, Lagana, & Gonzalez-Ramirez 1996).

Informing the Patient about Serious Illness

Family may want to protect an ill relative from knowing the seriousness or grave prognosis of an illness that the patient is suffering, based on the concern that patient's health may worsen if the poor prognosis is known. Information about the gravity of the illness is usually handled by a family spokesperson—often an older daughter or son (Paula, Lagana, & Gonzalez-Ramirez 1996).

Birth of a Child

Traditionally, men are not usually present at the delivery of a child. Female members in the family—such as the mother, mother-in-law, grandmothers, or elder sisters—assist and coach during labor. However, contemporary young couples may attend childbirth preparation classes together. These encourage active participation of the father, which is more and more accepted. Normal spontaneous vaginal delivery is preferred and elective caesarean delivery is feared because the surgery is viewed as life-threatening.

Various ethnic groups living in American society have been selected for a discussion of culture and healthcare in this chapter,. The intention has been to help healthcare providers be aware of the remarkable diversity that exists, and to provide some basic cultural knowledge that will lead to culturally competent care for these groups. Caution is needed, however, not to stereotype these groups. Every patient needs to be approached respectfully, and recognized for his or her individual beliefs and values.

References

Abu Gharbeih P (1993) Culture shock: Cultural norms influencing nursing in Jordan. Nursing and Healthcare 14:534–540

Afghani A, Abbott AV, Wiswell RA, Jaque SV, Gleckner C, Schroeder ET, Johnson CA (2004) Central adiposity, aerobic fitness, and blood pressure in premenopausal Hispanic women. International Journal of Sports Medicine 25:599–606

Artinian NT, Schim SM, Vander Wal JS, Nies MA (2004) Eating patterns and cardiovascular disease risk in a Detroit Mexican American population. Public Health Nursing 21:425–34

Bernstein L, Flannery J, Reynolds J (1993) Cancer in Italian migrant populations in the United States. IARC Science Publication 123:95–102

Black L (1996) Families of African origin: An overview. In: McGoldrick M, Giordano J, Pearce JK (eds) Ethnicity and Family Therapy. Guilford Press, New York, pp 57–65

Centers for Disease Control and Prevention (CDC) (2006) Trends in tuberculosis—United States, 2005. MMWR Morbidity and Mortality Weekly Report 55:305–8

Daley CM, Daley SM (2003) Care of American Indians and Alaska Natives. In: Bigby J (ed) Cross-cultural Medicine. American College of Physicians, Philadelphia, pp 95–128

Department of Health and Human Services (2001) Mental healthcare for American Indians and Alaska Natives. In: Mental Health: Culture, Race, and Ethnicity (a supplement to Mental Health: A Report to the Surgeon General). U.S. Public Health Service, Washington D.C. pp 77–104

Fernandez ES, South-Paul JE, Matheny SC (2003) Culture, race, and ethnicity issues in healthcare. In: Taylor RB (ed) Family Medicine: Principles and Practice. Springer, New York pp 17–23

Fitzgibon ML, Gapstur SM, Knight SJ (2004) Results of Mujeres Fellices por ser Saludabies: a dietary/breast health randomized clinical trial for Latino women. Annals of Behavioral Medicine 28(2):95–104

Garcia-Preto N (1996) Latino families: An overview. In: McGoldrick M, Giordano J, Pearce JK (eds) Ethnicity and Family Therapy. Guilford Press, New York, pp 141–154

Giordano J, McGoldrick M (1996) European families: An overview. In: McGoldrick M, Giordano J, Pearce JK (eds) Ethnicity and Family Therapy. Guilford Press, New York, pp 427–441

Glanville CL (2003) People of African American heritage. In: Purnell LD, Paulanka BJ (eds) Transcultural Healthcare: A Culturally Competent Approach, 2nd edn. F. A. Davis Company, Philadelphia, pp 40–53

Glazer N (1957) American Judaism.University of Chicago Press, Chicago

Goddard I (1990) An Afrocentric Model of Prevention for African-American High-risk Youth. Institute for the Advanced Study of Black Family Life and Culture, Oakland, California

Hammound MM, Siblani MK (2003) Care of Arab Americans and American Muslims. In: Bigby JA (ed) Cross-cultural Medicine. American College of Physicians, Philadelphia

Hillman SM (2003) People of Italian heritage. In: Purnell LD, Paulanka BJ (eds) Transcultural Healthcare: A Culturally Competent Approach, 2nd edn. F. A. Davis Company, Philadelphia, pp 205–217

Hostetler JA (1993) Amish Society, 4th edn. Johns Hopkins University Press, Baltimore, Maryland

Johnson JC, Slusar MB, Chaatre S, Johnsen P (2006) Perceptions of cultural competency among elderly African Americans. Ethnicity and Disease 16:778–85

Kitano HHL, Maki MT (1996) Continuity, change, and diversity: Counseling Asian Americans. In: Pedersen PB, Draguns JG, Lonner WJ, Trimble JE (eds) Counseling Across Cultures, 4th edn. Sage, Thousand Oaks, California, pp 124–145

Kramer J (1996) American Indians. In: Lioson JG, Diblle SL, Minarik PA (eds) Culture and Nursing Care: A Pocket Guide. UCSF Nursing Press, San Francisco

Kulwicki AD (2003) People of Arab heritage. In: Purnell LD, Paulanka BJ (eds) Transcultural Healthcare: A Culturally Competent Approach, 2nd edn. F. A. Davis Company, Philadelphia, pp 90–105

Maretzki TW, McDermott JF Jr. (1980) In McDermott JF Jr., Tseng WS, Maretzki TW (eds) People and cultures of Hawaii: A psychocultural profile (pp.24-52). Honolulu: University of Hawaii Press.

McGoldrick M (1982) Irish Families. In: McGoldrick M, Pearce JK, Giordano J (eds) Ethnicity and Family Therapy. The Guilford Press, New York, pp 310–339

Meleis AI (1996) Arab Americans. In: Lioson JG, Diblle SL, Minarik PA (eds) Culture and Nursing Care: A Pocket Guide. UCSF Nursing Press, San Francisco

Mittman IS, Bowie JV, Maman S (2007) Exploring the discourse between genetic counselors and orthodox Jewish community members related to reproductive genetic technology. Patient Education and Counseling 65:230–6

National Foundation for Jewish Genetic Diseases (2001) http://www.nfjgd.org/Factsheets/Fsindex.htm

Norton IM, Manson SM (1996) Research in American Indian and Alaska Native communities: Navigating the cultural universe of values and process. Journal of Consulting and Clinical Psychology 64:856–860

Oken D (1961) What to tell cancer patients: a study of medical attitudes. JAMA 175:1120–1128

Paula T, Lagana K, Gonzalez-Ramirez L (1996) Mexican Americans. In: Lioson JG, Diblle SL, Minarik PA (eds) Culture and Nursing Care: A Pocket Guide. UCSF Nursing Press, San Francisco

Poon AW, Gray KV, Franco GC, Cerruti DM, Schreck MA, Delgado ED (2003) Cultural competence: Serving Latino patients. Journal of Pediatric Orthopaedics 23:546–9

Rosner F (1993, July/August) Hospice, medical ethics and Jewish customs. American Journal of Hospice and Palliative Care 6–10

Selekman J (2003) People of Jewish heritage. In: Purnell LD, Paulanka BJ (eds) Transcultural Healthcare: A Culturally Competent Approach, 2nd edn. F. A. Davis Company, Philadelphia, pp 234–248

Snow L (1983) Traditional health beliefs and practice among lower class black American. Western Journal of Medicine 139:820–828

Stevers R (1976) A hair of the dog: Irish drinking and American stereotype. Pennsylvania State University Press, University Park, Pennsylvania

Stewart D, Johnson W, Saunders E (2006) Hypertension in back Americans as a special population: why so special? Current Cardiology Reports 8:405–10

Sutton C, Nose MA, B (1996) American Indian families: An overview. In: McGoldrick M, Giordano J, Pearce JK (eds) Ethnicity and Family Therapy. Guilford Press, New York, pp 31–44

Trimble JE, Fleming CM, Beauvais F, Jumper-Thurman P (1996) Essential cultural and social strategies for counseling Native American Indians. In: Pedersen PB, Draguns JG, Lonner WJ, Trimble JE (eds) Counseling Across Cultures, 4th edn. Sage, Thousand oaks, California, pp 177–209

Underwood S (1994) Increasing the participation of minorities and other at-risk groups in clinical trials. Innovations in Oncology Nursing 10:106

U. S. Bureau of the Census (1995) Statistical Abstract of the United States: The National Data Book. U. S. Census Bureau, Washington D.C.

U. S. Bureau of the Census (1999) Statistical Abstract of the United States: The National Data Book. U. S. Census Bureau, Washington D.C.

U. S. Bureau of the Census (2001) Profiles of general demographic characteristics: 2000 Census of Population and Housing—United States. U. S. Census Bureau, Washington D.C.

Welch M (2003) Care of Blacks and African Americans. In: Gigby J (ed) Cross-cultural Medicine American College of Physicians, Philadelphia pp 29–60

Wenger AFZ, Wenger MR (2003) The Amish. In: Purnell LD, Paulanka BJ (eds) Transcultural Healthcare: A Culturally Competent Approach, 2nd edn. F. A. Davis Company, Philadelphia, pp 54–72

Wilson SA (2003) People of Irish heritage. In: Purnell LD, Paulanka BJ (eds) Transcultural Healthcare: A Culturally Competent Approach, 2nd edn. F. A. Davis Company, Philadelphia

Zola IK (1983) Socio-medical inquires: Recollections, reflections, and reconsideration. Temple University Press, Philadelphia

Chapter 5
Culture and Medical Diseases

Culture-Related Perceptions of Certain Medical Diseases

Because of their poor prognosis and historically limited effectiveness of treatment, the diagnosis of certain medical diseases still carries substantial stigma or misunderstanding despite advances in medical knowledge and management. The following are some examples of diseases that are still associated with strong negative views or misconceptions as a result of cultural beliefs and that intensely influence patients' emotional lives as well as their illness or behavior.

Venereal Diseases, Including AIDS

Due to the fact that venereal diseases are usually associated with socially unsanctioned sexual behavior—such as prostitution, promiscuity, premarital intercourse, and extramarital affairs—venereal diseases are considered shameful in many societies. Patients will try to conceal them from other people—even from their own family members. Patients are hesitant to see physicians, so clinics may be set up in locations where visits will not be easily noticed by others.

Because of the devastating physical effects of AIDS, its association with drug abuse or homosexual behavior, and the possibility of contagion—either homosexually (in most Euro-American societies) or heterosexually (in Africa or Asian societies)—this condition has been particularly stigmatized. A great deal of denial about the prevalence, the need for treatment, and even the cause of the disease, still exists in some countries—even reaching the highest political levels.

In 2003, an estimated 1.2 million people in the United States were living with human immunodeficiency virus (HIV) infection. Among them, 47 percent were African-Americans, in spite of the fact that they accounted for only 11.9 percent of the total population of the United States. This shows that there are significant racial disparities in diagnosis of HIV/acquired immunodeficiency syndromes (AIDS) in the United State (Center for Disease Control and Prevention 2006).

As pointed out by Poindexter (2005), healthcare providers need to provide adequate attention and support not only to AIDS patients but also to their families in dealing with the matter of stigma, the complex management of the disease, caregiver stress, and issues related to spirituality and the meaning and of sickness and death.

Although the situation in the United States is improving as the prognosis for HIV infection improves, some physicians and dentists have been reluctant to come in contact with—and provide care for—patients with this disorder. A survey of Asian versus Caucasian dentists practicing in New York City revealed that Asian dentists expressed significantly more negative attitudes toward—and unwillingness to treat—HIV-positive patients than did Caucasian dentists (Raphael, Kunzel, Sadowsky 1996). A study of senior dental students at the University of Iowa found a wide range of comfort with regard to the treatment of patients with special needs and other vulnerable populations, yet no more than 60 percent of these students were willing to treat HIV/AIDS patients (Kuthy, McQuistan, Riniker, Heller & Qian 2005).

The stigma of AIDS can lead to policies based on fear, disproportionate to a given society's needs. This is occurring in China, where massive resources have been devoted to managing the disease, even while the burden of disease from HIV remains low. If similar resources were devoted to tobacco-control measures, the effect on public health could be huge. Treatment for such common conditions as tuberculosis, hypertension, or cataracts may require payment in the same settings where HIV treatment is free (Hesketha 2007).

Cancer

Patients of varying backgrounds react differently to having a potentially fatal disease. Individual personality, family background, age, and gender are some of the factors that influence a patient's reaction to cancer. Ethnic and cultural factors can contribute importantly to different reactions.

For example, to study cross-ethnic differences among cancer patients' attitudes toward their disease, Ali, Khalil, and Yousef (1993) compared the results of structured interviews of American patients in a Midwestern hospital with those of Egyptian patients at a hospital in Cairo, Egypt. Analysis of the responses revealed five categories of attitudes among the American patients, including (in order) fighting spirit and adaptation, fear/anxiety/disbelief, hope, passivity in planning, and faith. Among Egyptian patients, seven categories emerged in the following order: stoicism and fatalism, dependency, compliance with the medical regimen, anxiety/fear/insecurity, powerlessness, hope and optimism, and family support. This study illustrated how patients with different ethnic backgrounds from different societies (possibly with different medical realities) vary in their reactions to cancer. American patients, based on their cultural attitudes, mostly held views of adaptation and hope. Egyptian patients, based on their philosophical orientation, maintained more fatalistic and powerless views.

Breast Cancer

Breast cancer is unique in the sense that the breast is a part of the female anatomy with emotion-laden symbolic connotations involving sexuality and nurturance. The disease is also potentially fatal and treatment is potentially mutilating. Among immigrant groups and women from traditional cultures, breast cancer may be shrouded in fears and myths that go far beyond an objective medical understanding of the disease. These women may fail to access available breast-screening services, and present with advanced symptoms. Structural barriers preventing early diagnosis and treatment include such factors as poor health insurance, distance to medical facilities, and inability to take time off from work. Organizational barriers include the necessity to navigate complex healthcare systems and to interact with medical staff who may relate with less than optimal cultural sensitivity. Socio-cultural barriers include fatalism, mistrust of cancer treatments, and the fear of becoming a burden on family members. These barriers can often preclude proactive breast screening or rapid response to symptoms, even when breast cancer awareness is rather high. Moreover, in Muslim and other traditional societies, women's decisions are controlled by men, who may be unaware of or disapprove of breast screening. Cultural competence training can help healthcare providers work with these at-risk women (Remennick 2006).

Leprosy

Leprosy is a rare but serious mycobacterial infection. The infection results in chronic dermatitis and peripheral nerve involvement. Due to the visible malformation of the face or hands, plus its long history without effective treatment in the past, leprosy is still stigmatized as a particularly terrible disease in many societies, and contact with such patients is shunned (Heijnders 2004). Therefore, in the past century, leprosy patients were usually isolated from the community. In Hawaii, one isolated region of a small neighbor island has been used as the leprosy sanctuary that isolated an infected person for life. Leprosy is uncommon in developed countries nowadays, but it is important for physicians to have a high index of suspicion of foreign-born immigrant patients (particularly from tropical areas) with chronic dermatitis and peripheral nerve sensory loss (Boggild, Correia, Keysonte & Kain 2004). For physicians to take into account the quality of life of the patient, they need to consider not only the medical aspects of the disorder and therapeutic options, but also the psychological and social aspects of the disorder (Chaturvedi, Singh & Gupta 2005).

Pulmonary Tuberculosis

Before the appearance of effective antibiotics for treatment, pulmonary tuberculosis ran a chronic and fatal course. People were afraid of this contagious disease and patients tended to keep it secret from others. In China, it was called the *life disease*, meaning that once it was contracted, the patient would suffer for a lifetime and die early because there was no cure. After the availability of effective antibiotics and thorough screening tests, the prevalence of pulmonary tuberculosis declined sharply in most developed societies. However, it is still prevalent in developing societies where nutrition is not good, hygiene is poor, and people tend to live in crowded settings. Compulsory physical exams for immigrants, and provision of appropriate treatment for those patients screened positive, are especially important from the public health perspective. Healthcare providers face cultural stigmas attached to this disease when they encourage active treatment (Car & Partridge 2004).

Epilepsy

Folk healers have attributed a number of unusual causes to epilepsy, such as the patient being possessed by evil spirits or the illness being the result of an ancestor's immoral behavior. In traditional Chinese medicine, the observation that many epileptic patients have saliva coming out of their mouth was interpreted as a morbid condition due to excessive *yin* element because saliva belongs to *yin*. Therefore, the proper management of epilepsy consisted of taking adequate *yang* element—such as ginger and spicy food.

In the United Kingdom, Ismail, Wright, Rhodes, and Small (2005) interviewed South Asian epileptic patients (who were Muslims, Sikhs, and Hindus) about their view of epilepsy. They found that over half of the responders attributed their illness to fate and the will of God. They commonly turned to traditional healers in search of better health.

Knowing that socio-cultural attitudes continue to have a negative impact on the management of epilepsy in many African countries and in a few advanced countries, Nubukpoet, Preux, Clement, et al. (2003) compared attitudes toward epilepsy in France with that in two African nations—Togo and Benin. The epileptic patients were interviewed using a questionnaire about their beliefs, knowledge, attitudes, and practices regarding their disease. The researchers found out that the number of people who believed in supernatural causes of epilepsy was higher in Togo and Benin while the number of people attributing the diseases to social causes (such as stress) was higher in France. Few epileptic patients in France thought that the disease was contagious, in comparison to patients in both Togo and Benin. Some foods were forbidden in Togo and Benin because of superstitious beliefs that consumption of these foods would cause seizures. More patients in France were aware of the relationship between epilepsy and alcohol, drug abuse, and cerebral injury. Epileptic patients in France were more likely to consult a physician and use medical drugs for the treatment than their counterparts in Togo and Benin. Epileptic patients in Togo often complained of social exclusion.

In a study of the perception of epilepsy in Seoul, South Korea, persons were randomly selected and interviewed by telephone regarding public awareness, knowledge, and attitudes toward epilepsy. Almost half the population believed that epilepsy is heritable and untreatable. Marriage of their children to an epileptic person, childbearing by women with epilepsy, and employing a person with epilepsy were opposed by more than half of the respondents (Choi-Kwon, Park, Lee, Park, Lee, Cheon, Youn, Lee & Chung 2004). Thus, social stigma toward epilepsy is still prominent in some cultures.

Malaria

Although it is quite commonly understood that malaria is spread by a particular type of mosquito, and that control of this mosquito is the essential way to prevent the transmission of such disease, this understanding is not necessarily shared by some peoples at risk (Agyepong 1992; Morgan & Figueroa-Munoz 2005). For example, people of the Ga-Adangbe tribe in southern Ghana, Africa—who recognize a syndrome they call *asra*, consisting of fever, chills, headaches, bodily pains, and so on—did not recognize that this condition (actually malaria) was caused by the bite of a mosquito. Almost all the people in the community believed that it was caused by contact with excessive external heat—especially from sunlight—but also from cooking, burning charcoal, and standing too close to a fire. They interpreted that accumulated heat upset the body balance, affecting the blood. They believed that it was a condition that could not be avoided because they had to work outdoors in the harsh sunlight. If they suffered from the condition, they were cared for at home—rarely in the hospital.

In North America, immigrants are frequent travelers to malaria-prone areas, visiting friends and relatives. Eliciting cultural beliefs about malaria increases the opportunity to provide effective preventative measures (Bacaner, Stauffer, Boulware, Walker & Keystone 2004).

Dementia

Dementia is a disorder characterized by an incremental loss of memory and intellectual functioning. Usually there is a gradual onset and, in the beginning, the disorder may not be recognized by family—particularly if the affected individual is not working and is not expected to perform complex tasks. As dementia progresses, becoming more severe, the individual is unable to perform basic tasks of daily living, including such things as taking care of financial matters, preparing food, maintaining normal hygiene, dressing appropriately, and avoiding harm. These tasks will then require others to manage daily living for the affected person—often family members or, in some settings, institutions designed to take care the disabled.

While biological factors are primary in the development and phenomenology of dementia, social roles and expectations determine how disabling and disruptive this condition will be. Furthermore, the response of family and caregivers has significant cultural determinants. The roles and expectations of the individual, who is usually elderly, influence when the family recognizes and becomes concerned about the demented relative's behavior. Culture affects the degree to which family members desire or feel obligated to care for their loved one.

Caregiving for a demented individual can be very stressful. A great deal of time and effort may be required. The demented individual may not be able to express appreciation to the caregiver. Although not always the case, the personality may have changed, and there may be frequent and repetitive demands, outbursts of anger, or cries for help. The stress of caregiving can be potentially overwhelming and cause depression. The perception of stress and reward in caregiving varies in different cultures.

A number of studies have compared white and African-American responses to caregiving for those with dementia. African-Americans often delayed seeking medical help for a relative with Alzheimer's Disease for years, and the delay was unrelated to educational level (Clark, Kutner, Goldstein, Peterson-Hazen, Garner, Zhang & Bowles 2005). African-American caregivers were more likely to turn to religion and to use denial to help cope. Whites were more likely to use humor and acceptance as coping styles. Although whites had more financial resources, African-Americans were less burdened (Kosberg, Kaufman, Burgio, Leeper & Sun 2007). In another study, blacks were found to overrate, while whites underrated the cognitive abilities of the affected individual (Burns, Nichols, Graney, Martindale-Adams & Lummus 2006).

For Alzheimer's patients, memory and behavioral problems correlated with increasing depressive symptomatology in black caregivers, but not whites, however. Thus, the impact of the severity of dementia is not homogeneous across a race (Williams 2005.)

In a large, multi-site study, African-American caregivers reported much less stress than Caucasian caregivers. They had lower anxiety, were bothered less by the behavior of the demented individual, used psychotropic medications less, perceived more benefits from caregiving, and endorsed greater religious coping and participation. All this was despite African-American caregivers' lower socioeconomic status (Haley, Gitlin, Wisniewski, Mahoney, Coon, Winter, Corcoran, Schinfeld, & Ory 2004).

Fewer studies compare the caregiving roles of other cultural groups. In general, whites experience more stress and are faster to recognize dementia and institutionalize an affected relative. Other groups are more likely to view dementia as a normal phenomenon—part of the aging process (e.g., Hinton, Guo, Hillygus & Levkoff 2000). White caregivers are the most likely to be spouses and less likely to be children, in comparison with other groups.

To summarize, the onset and prevalence of dementia are much more strongly influenced by biology than culture, although cultural factors influence the degree of disability—particularly in the milder forms of dementia. Cultural factors are much more powerful in determining caregiver issues, however.

Case Vignette

A 66-year old, retired Samoan immigrant had recently developed end-stage renal disease, secondary to diabetic nephropathy. His vision was poor, and he had experienced increasing short-term memory problems over the last year or two, diagnosed as a mild dementia. He lived at home with his wife and teenage daughter. He also had an elder daughter, who was married and the mother of a toddler. He had had a successful career, and he was a somewhat demanding man, whose wife was rather timid by comparison.

He now required maintenance hemodialysis, and his dietary restrictions increased, as did the number of his medications. As he came to terms with all this, and not wanting to overburden his wife, he decided that his two daughters should stay home as much as possible to help attend to his needs. This meant that his younger daughter needed to come home straight from school, not participate in any school activities, and not spend any afterschool time with friends. His elder daughter was living in another state, where her husband was employed. She was told to move back to the parents' home. This meant she would be living apart from her husband as long as the father needed her.

Both daughters were unhappy at this turn of events, but accepted that this was their obligation and did not protest. The father cried when the medical staff asked how much this would disrupt his daughters' lives, but he did not relent in his demands. He stated, "It is the Samoan way (fa'a Samoa)."

In this case, the medical staff was quite disturbed at what they thought was an unfair caregiver burden being placed on the daughters, even though the daughters did not protest or complain. If the daughters were more acculturated to American culture, the conflict caused by the father's demands might have resulted in significant distress and emotional symptoms. At that point, the medical staff could have reasonably searched for a culturally appropriate solution—or, if necessary, one that challenged the patient's demands because of the particular circumstances. A physician, social worker, or mental health worker—individually, or (better) as a team—could have approached the patient, pointing out that life in America is not the same as a small island in Samoa where people can move easily between villages. Arrangements could have been made to structure the patient's environment and help support the wife's caregiving role in such a way that the patient would feel as secure as possible. The authority of the medical staff could have been invoked to insist upon the best course of action for the family.

Culture and Prevalence of Certain Medical Disorders

Although many diseases are predominantly biomedical in nature—with biological origins that are genetic, infectious, traumatic, metabolic, neoplastic, and so on—there are many medical disorders that are influenced indirectly by the patient's life style, which in turn is shaped by socioeconomic conditions or cultural beliefs. As a result, there are remarkable differences in how often such disorders occur and are observed in certain societies. It is impossible to list all such medical disorders, so we will present only a few of the more well-studied examples to illustrate how social and cultural factors influence the prevalence of medical disorders.

Coronary Heart Disease

Coronary heart disease has multiple etiological or risk factors, including hereditary, elevated lipids, hypertension, diabetes, smoking, and so on. The emotional life, or lifestyle, of the patients affects these risk factors, and also influences the incidence and outcome of the disease.

For example, coronary heart disease morbidity and mortality are more prevalent in blacks than whites in the United States. A recent study found clear differences among subgroups of blacks. Immigrant blacks had better coronary risk profiles and lower proportions of persons with metabolic syndrome and other heart disease-related conditions. The authors of this study concluded that future studies of diet and health should consider cultural differences within the black population to better understand and reduce overall health disparities in the United States (Lancaster, Watts & Dixon 2006).

In general, however, most studies have found a higher prevalence of coronary disease in immigrants undergoing acculturation stress. A large, multiethnic study found that time in the United States raises the risk of coronary calcification in Chinese and blacks, and that this is independent of the traditional coronary risk factors of smoking, diabetes, body mass index, lipid profile, and hypertension (Diez Roux, Detrano, Jackson, Jacobs, Schreiner, Shea & Szklo 2005).

In their numerous studies (Marmot, Syme, Kanga, Kato, Cohen & Belsky 1975; Marmot & Syme 1976), Marmot and colleagues have examined the epidemiology of coronary heart disease, hypertension, and stroke among 11,900 men of Japanese ancestry living in California, Hawaii, and Japan, respectively. The aim was to identify the influence of nongenetic factors on these three groups for the occurrence of cardiovascular disease. They found that there is a gradient in the occurrence of coronary heart disease among the three groups, with the lowest rate in Japan, intermediate in Hawaii, and the highest in California. The influence of other risk factors commonly associated with high coronary heart disease, such as hypertension, diet, smoking, weight, blood sugar, and serum cholesterol levels was examined. It was found that the gradient in the incidence of coronary heart disease could not be explained fully by the presence of these risk factors. Instead, the incidence of coronary heart disease was found to be related to the degree of adherence to traditional Japanese culture. The closer the adherence to traditional values and customs was, the lower the incidence of coronary heart disease became.

A recent study confirmed these original observations. The incidence of coronary heart disease in Japan has remained low despite increases in coronary risk factors—including major dietery changes. This is known as the *Japanese paradox*. Genetic factors do not explain this, because migrating Japanese develop rates of coronary disease close to that of the host country (Sekikawa, Ueshima, Kadowaki, El-Saed, Okamura, Takamiya, Kashiwagi, Edmundowicz, Murata, Sutton-Tyrrell, Maegawa, Evans, Kita & Kuller 2007).

Cervical Cancer

The exact cause of cervical cancer is still unknown—believed to be multi-factorial in origin—and there is a strong suspicion that a viral infection is often implicated. Various studies have shown that cervical cancer is rare in nuns and common in prostitutes. It is extremely uncommon among Jewish, Mormon, and Seventh Day Adventist women. These findings suggest that the occurrence of cervical cancer has to do with women's sexual behavior. Women with cervical cancer are more likely to have experienced early commencement of coitus, early marriage, multiple sexual partners, and multiple marriages. It was originally thought that a woman's sexual behavior alone could determine her risk of cervical cancer. But, based on the observation that the incidence of cervical cancer is very high in Latin America, Skegg, Corwin, Pau, and Doll (1982) speculated that a women's risk of getting the disease depends less on her sexual behavior than on that of her husband or male partner. They postulated three types of society in terms of sexual behavior of men and women. In Type A, both men and women are strongly discouraged from pre- or extramarital relations. This is exemplified by Mormons or Seventh Day Adventists, who have the lowest prevalence of cervical cancer. In Type B, only women are strongly discouraged from extramarital sexual relations but men are expected to have many (especially with prostitutes). This is seen in many Latin American societies, which have a high incidence of cervical cancer. In Type C, both men and women have several sexual partners during their lives. This pattern occurs in the United Kingdom and the United States, yet there is a declining rate of cervical cancer. This may be due to the changing patterns of sexual behavior, with less recourse to prostitutes in a more permissive society.

Obesity

Obesity refers to an excessive percentage of body fat. The commonly used measure of excessive body weight is the Body Mass Index (BMI). However, there is controversy over the universal application of BMI as a measure of obesity because BMI cut-off points do not always accurately reflect morbidity and mortality. This is due to the fact that ethnic/racial groups have different body types and body tissue compositions. In some eras, obesity has been viewed as representing wealth, beauty, and health by some cultures. Today, however, it is medically considered to be an unhealthy condition—a risk factor for cardiovascular disease, diabetes, and other disorders.

Obesity has become a world-wide phenomenon. More people are now overweight than underweight (Okpaku 2006). It is estimated that 300 million people in the world are obese. In certain parts of the world—such as the Pacific Islands, some parts of Eastern Europe, the Middle East, and China—the rate of obesity has increased threefold since 1980. In the United States, obesity has nearly doubled since 1980, with the rate of increase greatest for African-Americans and Hispanics (Cossrow & Falkner 2004). Sixty percent of the population is now overweight (Wyatt, Winters & Dubbert 2006). Within most countries, there are decreased physical activity levels, increased television viewing, and a tendency to consume high caloric food—resulting in more overweight youth and a propensity of carrying that extra weight into adulthood.

People of certain societies (such as Polynesians) tend to have heavier, stockier builds than those of other societies (such as some Asians) who tend to have a slender body habitus. Under the influence of changing habits that include high fat, high calorie food and a lack of physical exercise, the prevalence of obesity has been soaring among most ethnicities. In South Korea, however, cultural factors seem to have caused significant increases in obesity despite changing dietary habits (Kim, Moon & Popkin 2000). It is no wonder that obesity is regarded as a medical-social-cultural disorder.

Culture, Food Intake, and Medical Disorders

To consume food is essential—not only to sustain life, but also to satisfy psychological needs, facilitate social relations, and follow culturally shaped lifestyles. Therefore, there are remarkably different food-intake patterns among different societies. Some culturally-related food habits have direct implications for the occurrence of certain medical disorders. Some examples will be presented here to illustrate this point.

Rickets occurs at a much higher rate among Asian people living in the United Kingdom than the local white population. This may be due in part to a deficiency of vitamin D in the Asian vegetarian dietary habits practiced there (Stroud 1963). The habit of chewing certain nuts—practiced by people in Micronesia, aboriginal people in the Philippines or Malaysia, and others—may contribute to the occurrence of lip cancer.

Perhaps the most dramatic instance of culturally related disease caused by a food habit is the rare and unique disease of *Kuru*. *Kuru* is a neuro-degenerative disease found only in the Okapa District of the Eastern Highlands Province of Papua, New Guinea. The disease usually begins with trouble walking, and causes steady deterioration with dementia and inevitable death. In the past, local people believed that the patients were cursed. However, it was eventually related to their food-intake patterns. After a death, relatives of the deceased would eat the dead person's brains (to keep the deceased relative's soul and vitality within themselves). The infectious agent—a *prion*—then passed on to those who ate the brains. This practice of cannibalism stopped by 1960, but due to very long incubation periods, cases are still being reported (Collinge, Whitfield, McKintosh, Beck, Mead, Thomas & Alpers 2006).

References

Agyepong IA (1992) Malaria: Ethnomedical perceptions and practice in an Adangbe farming community and implications for control. Social Science and Medicine 35:131–137

Ali NS, Khalil HZ, Yousef W (1993) A comparison of American and Egyptian cancer patients' attitudes and unmet needs. Cancer Nursing 16(3):193–203

Bacaner N, Stauffer B, Boulware DR, Walker PF, Keystone JS (2004) Travel medicine considerations for North American immigrants visiting friends and relatives. JAMA 291:2856–64

Boggiled AK, Correia JD, Keystone JS, Kain KC (2004) Leprosy in Toronto: An analysis of 184 imported cases. Canadian Medical Association Journal 170:55–59

Burns R, Nichols LO, Graney MJ, Martindale-Adams J Lummus A (2006) Cognitive abilities of Alzheimer's patients: Perceptions of Black and White caregivers. Int J Aging Hum Dev 62:209–19

Car J, Partridge MR (2004) Crosscultural communication in those with airway diseases. Chronic Respiratory Diseases 1:153–160

Centers for Disease Control and Prevention (CDC) (2006) Racial/ethnic disparities in diagnoses of HIV/AIDS – 33 states, 2001–2004. MMWR Morbidity and Mortality Report 55(5):121–125

Chaturvedi SK, Singh G, Gupta N (2005) Stigma experience in skin disorders: An Indian perspective. Dermatology Clinics, 23(4):635–642

Choi-Kwon S, Park KA, Lee HJ, Park MS, Lee CH, Cheon SE, Youn MH, Lee SK, Chung CK (2004) Familiarity with, knowledge of, and attitudes toward epilepsy in residents of Seoul, South Korea. Acta Neurologica Scandinavica 110(1):39–45

Clark PC, Kutner NG, Goldstein FC, Peterson-Hazen S, Garner V, Zhang R, Bowles T (2005) Impediments to timely diagnosis of Alzheimer's disease in African Americans. J Am Geriatr Soc 53:2012–7.

Collinge J, Whitfield J, McKintosh E, Beck J, Mead S, Thomas DJ, Alpers MP (2006) Kuru in the 21st century–an acquired human prion disease with very long incubation periods. Lancet 367(9528):2068–74

Cossrow N, Falkner B (2004) Race/ethnic issues in obesity and obesity-related comorbidities. Journal of Clinical Endocrinology and Metabolism 89:2590–4

Diez Roux AV, Detrano R, Jackson S, Jacobs DR, Schreiner PJ, Shea S, Szklo, M (2005) Acculturation and socioeconomic position as predictors of coronary calcification in a multiethnic sample. Circulation 112:1557–65

Haley WE, Gitlin LN, Wisniewski SR, Mahoney DF, Coon DW, Winter L, Corcoran M, Schinfeld S Ory M (2004) Well-being, appraisal, and coping in African-American and Caucasian dementia caregivers: findings from the REACH study. Aging Ment Health 8:316–29

Heijnders ML (2004) The dynamics of stigma in leprosy. International Journal of Leprosy and Other Mycobacterial Diseases 72:437–47

Hesketha T (2007) HIV/AIDS in China: the numbers problem. Lancet 369(9562):621–623

Hinton L, Guo Z, Hillygus J Levkoff S (2000) Working with culture: a qualitative analysis of barriers to the recruitment of Chinese-American family caregivers for dementia research. Journal of Cross Cultural Gerontology 15:119–37

Ismail H, Wright J, Rhodes P, Small N (2005) Religious beliefs about causes and treatment of epilepsy. British Journal of General Practice 55(510):26–31

Kim S, Moon S, Popkin BM (2000) The nutrition transition in South Korea. American Journal of Clinical Nutrition 71:44–53

Kosberg JI, Kaufman AV, Burgio LD, Leeper JD, Sun F (2007) Family caregiving to those with dementia in rural Alabama: Racial similarities and differences. J Aging Health 19:3–21

Kuthy RA, McQuistan MR, Riniker KJ, Heller KE, Qian F (2005) Students' comfort level in treating vulnerable populations and future willingness to treat: Results prior to extramural participation. Journal of Dental Education 69(12):1307–1314

Lancaster KJ, Watts SO Dixon LB (2006) Dietary intake and risk of coronary heart disease differ among ethnic subgroups of black Americans. Journal of Nutrition 136:446–51

Marmot MG, Syme SL (1976) Acculturation and coronary heart disease in Japanese Americans. American Journal of Epidemiology 104:225–247

Marmot MG, Syme SL, Kagan A, Kato H, Cohen JB, Belsky J (1975) Epidemiological studies of coronary heart disease and stroke in Japanese men living in Japan, Hawaii and California: Prevalence of coronary and hypertensive heart disease and associated risk factor. American Journal of Epidemiology 102:514–525

Morgan M, Figueroa-Munoz JI (2005) Barriers to uptake and adherence with malaria prophylaxis by the African community in London, England: Focus group study. Ethnicity and Health 10:355–72

Nubukpo P, Preux PM, Clement JP, Houinato D, Tuillas M, Aubreton C, Radji A, Grunitzky EK, Avode G, Tapie P (2003) Comparison of sociocultural attitudes towards epilepsy in Limousin (France), in Togo and in Benin (Africa). Medicine Tropicale (Marseilles) 63(2):143–50

Okpaku S (2006) Culture and Obesity: World's New Trend and Problems. The Proceeding of the First World Congress of Cultural Psychiatry S-II-20

Poindexter CC (2005) Working with HIV-affected culturally diverse families. In: Congress EP, Gonzalerz MJ (eds) Multicultural perspectives in working with families. Springer, New York pp 311–338

Raphael KG, Kunzel C, Sadowsky D (1996) Difference between Asian-American and white American dentist students in attitudes toward treatment of HIV-positive patients. AIDS Education and Prevention 8(2):155–164

Remennick L (2006) The challenge of early breast cancer detection among immigrant and minority women in multicultural societies. The Breast Journal 12 (Suppl 1): S103–S110

Sekikawa A, Ueshima H, Kadowaki T, El-Saed A, Okamura T, Takamiya T, Kashiwagi A, Edmundowicz D, Murata K, Sutton-Tyrrell K, Maegawa H, Evans RW, Kita Y, Kuller LH (2007) Less subclinical atherosclerosis in Japanese men in Japan than in White men in the United States in the post-World War II birth cohort. American Journal of Epidemiology 165:617–24

Sich D (1979) Naeng: Geggegnung mit einer volkskrankheit in der modernen frauen aerztlichen sprech-stunde in Korea (Encounter with a folk illness during modern gynecolgocal consultations in Korea). Curare: Zeitschrift fur Ethnomedizin und Trans-kulturelle Psychiatrie 2:87–96 (Reviewed in Transcultual Psychiatric Research Review, 18:45–46 [1981] by Tobler AB)

Skegg DCG, Corwin PA, Pau C Doll R (1982) Importance of the male factor in cancer of the cervix. Lancet 2:581–583

Stroud CE (1963) Nutritional problem in the immigrant population in London. Proceeding of the Nutrition Society 22:153–158

Williams IC (2005) Emotional health of black and white dementia caregivers: a contextual examination. The Journals of Gerontology (Series B) Psychological Sciences and Social Sciences 60:287–295

Wyatt SB, Winters KP, Dubbert PM (2006) Overweight and obesity: prevalence, consequences, and causes of a growing public health problem. American Journal of Medical Science 331:166–74

Chapter 6
Culture and Mental Disorders

Cultural Aspects of Psychiatric Issues in the Care of Patients

Although this book is written primarily for health professionals in a broad sense—including physicians of various specialties, nurses, social workers, and other health-related workers—this chapter will focus specifically on care of patients whose problems include psychological or psychiatric issues to a greater or lesser degree. Many patients, whose problems are primarily psychiatric, are taken care of by nonpsychiatric physicians and other healthcare professionals. This can involve patients who initiate their help-seeking with primary care providers, those who develop psychiatric problems in the course of being treated for other conditions, those who do not have easy access to mental health providers, and those whose problems are not so complex that the primary providers feel the need to refer for adequate treatment to be achieved. Therefore, providing culturally appropriate and competent care for such psychiatric patients is a worthwhile and challenging task for physicians and other healthcare workers.

Cultural issues influence psychiatric problems to an extent that is usually more than areas of medicine that are predominantly biological in nature. This is because culture significantly impacts thought, emotion, behavior, and illness-related behavior—it has a strong influence on how people experience and manifest emotional problems, present psychiatric symptoms, and seek professional help.

How cultural factors influence patients who are suffering from psychiatric problems can be elaborated from different viewpoints, including symptom manifestation, help-seeking behaviors, clinical assessment, and treatment approaches.

Psychological Problems: Normality versus Pathology

For many medical conditions, it is not difficult to distinguish the boundary between normal and pathological. A bone fracture is a bone fracture, hepatitis is hepatitis, and pneumonia is pneumonia. When bone, liver, or lungs, for example, show signs of abnormality in conjunction with clinical symptoms, such is considered clearly pathological. There are also many areas of medicine, however, where the boundary between normal and abnormal is not so clear—such as blood pressure or cholesterol levels. Culture can conceivably play a role in these determinations, but a minor one if any. These conditions are in contrast to those where thoughts, emotions, or behaviors are the primary areas of concern. At what point is an active, energetic child considered pathologically hyperactive? How much alcohol can a person drink before an alcohol abuse problem is considered? The boundary between normality and pathology for mental health problems and psychiatric disorders is not absolute and varies with the contextual situation—culture being a particularly strong influence on where the boundary is set.

To distinguish normality from pathology, four approaches have been described (Offer & Sabshin, 1974). They are professional definition, deviation from the mean, assessment of function, and social definition.

Professional Definition

This approach takes the view that normality or pathology can be clearly differentiated by the nature of the phenomenon itself, and the judgment can be made by trained professionals. In general medicine, the occurrence of bleeding or a bone fracture is judged by the professionals to be pathological and in need of medical care by the nature of the condition. Likewise, in psychiatry, if a person talks to nonexistent people, claims to be hearing the voice of a spaceman, or eats his or her own feces, he or she will be professionally judged to be suffering from a pathological mental condition. This approach maintains that certain conditions (manifested as signs or symptoms) are absolutely pathological in nature. A diagnosis can be made on such a condition that is universally applicable—beyond cultural boundaries. Organic brain disorders—such as severe dementia or a delirious state, or a severe psychotic condition with very pathological thought disorders or disorganized behavior—tend to be easily diagnosed by experts without too much doubt, even cross-culturally.

However, caution is needed clinically to make the diagnosis of many psychiatric disorders. An example is the differentiation between dementia and pseudo-dementia. The latter refers to a person manifesting a dementia-like mental condition due to depression. An elderly patient who suffers from depression may lose interest in carrying out daily activities, including communicating with others, and may appear to be clinically suffering from dementia with a disturbance in memory. In fact, there may be no actual loss of memory or intellectual abilities, but instead the pathology is a depressed mood. Cultural factors can contribute to the likelihood of making the wrong diagnosis. This may happen if the clinician does not share the same language with the patient, and misinterpretations can occur with regard to mood and executive mental function. Even if the language is the same, misunderstandings and misinterpretations can occur when the meaning of what is said is influenced by cultural context. It is therefore important for a clinician not to automatically assume that understanding occurs if there are cultural differences with the patient.

Deviation from the Mean

This approach relies on mathematical measurement and obtained data and uses a range of deviation from the mean to distinguish between normal and abnormal. For example, hypertension, anemia, obesity, or subnormal intelligence are conditions that use certain scales and measurements to define normality. A pathological condition is diagnosed when the measurement goes a defined distance beyond the average range. The concept of the mean is universal, yet the range of deviation from the mean that is considered within normal limits often needs adjustment for different populations. This is notably true, for example, when personality is assessed by using questionnaires cross-culturally. The cutting point for defining behavior disorders, as measured by questionnaires, is another area that deserves careful cross-cultural adjustment. Determining the amount of drinking (or other substance use) that is excessive is another situation that needs biological, social, and cultural adjustments.

Assessment of Function

Whether a person has a healthy lung or not can be assessed by lung capacity and their ability to perform the function of respiration from the perspective of physiology. As with regard to mental disorders, this approach considers the effect of thoughts, feelings, or behavior on function. Whether the condition provides (healthy) function or (unhealthy) dysfunction for the individual is the basis for the judgment of normality versus pathology.

The assessment of memory is a good example. Its disturbance is determined by the extent to which a person can retain the obtained information and reproduce it usefully through recollection. If a person living in an urban setting cannot recall the street number of his own house, or the name of the street where he lives, and, thus, does not know how to return home, then memory is seen to be clearly impaired because it is so dysfunctional. In contrast, if a man living in a remote rural area, where street numbers are not significant, does not recall his own number, he may not be considered memory-impaired if he knows where his village is located, how his home looks, and how to find his way home. Thus, it is the purpose and function of memory that needs to be considered, rather than arbitrary information that can be recalled. When a clinician performs a mental status examination, memory is often tested by having the patient repeat random digits or recall three objects after a few minutes. The diagnosis of memory impairment is not on the basis of poor performance on these tests per se, but because poor performance correlates with functionally meaningful memory impairment involving daily activities.

Another example is outward behavior. Generally speaking, openly aggressive behavior that frequently disturbs the family, neighbors, or society will be perceived by the family or community as dysfunctional, and therefore pathological. On the other hand, quiet, seclusive, and asocial behavior—if it does not cause any problems to the surrounding people—may not be considered dysfunctional, and thus not labeled as pathological. Culture strongly influences the degree to which a society tolerates aggressive behavior on the one hand, and is accepting of quiet, seclusive behavior on the other. Studies have shown that the evaluation of the behavior of hyperactive children by clinicians varies greatly among different cultures. In other words, behavior tends to be judged primarily by its impact on the individual, others, and the environment from a functional point of view.

Social Definition

This approach utilizes social and cultural judgment in deciding whether behavior is normal or pathological. The decision is subject to the social knowledge and cultural attitudes found among the members of the society. Thus, the conclusion is subjective and collectively made. For instance, women wearing shorts and halter tops in warm weather is common, normal behavior in many countries—even going topless is quite acceptable in some societies—but such behavior would be considered unacceptably deviant in Islamic societies, even in very hot weather. Continuing to live with one's parents after age 30 may be interpreted as reflecting a dependency problem in American society, but may be regarded as natural and ordinary in Filipino society. To speak out against authority figures (such as parents, teachers, or the police) may be regarded as acceptable—even brave—behavior in a democratic society, but may be judged as antisocial in an autocratic society. The judgments made by a society may vary greatly, depending on its customs, beliefs, and values. In general, among all mental functions, social behavior tends to be assessed and defined predominantly by socio-culturally influenced judgments.

It is important for a clinician to be aware of which of the above approaches is being utilized in making a clinical judgment, to recognize the limitations of each approach, and to make whatever adjustments are necessary in putting together the final assessment.

Presentation of Problems and Clinical Assessment

In the field of medicine, medical information is gathered to make a *diagnosis*. The sources of medical information can be a patient's description of symptoms, the course of the illness, signs observed or detected through physical examination, or laboratory data obtained through testing. Thus, the patient contributes only part of the information needed for making a diagnosis. Furthermore, medical diagnosis is based on the assumption that there exist certain kinds of disease entities that are characterized by certain clusters of signs and symptoms, and can be categorized by certain diagnostic criteria. The gathered information is fitted to the diagnostic criteria for any recognized or classified disease entity. In other words, making a medical diagnosis involves trying to put information into existing pigeon holes. Once the diagnosis is made, a treatment plan can be carried out, and the course of the disease can be predicted—including the responses to the medicine prescribed. The cultural impact on the process of medical diagnosis is only partial. It is mainly related to how the patient makes complaints and describes symptoms.

To understand and treat mental disorders, however, other facts about the patient become particularly important. A clinician needs to know in detail not only about how the problems started, and how they are coped with, but also the information about the patient's personal life, family, personality, and behavior patterns. This includes how the patient perceives things, interprets and understands the things he observes, and what beliefs form from these cognitions. In other words, it is a process of understanding the patient from a broader perspective, including past and present, individual and family, intrapsychic and interpersonal, and conscious and unconscious. It is not a process focused merely on symptom complaints, but on the context within which the problems were encountered and developed. Even the symptoms need to be evaluated according to the patient's understanding, motivation, and functioning in making such complaints. All of these factors are influenced by the cultural background of the patient. Furthermore, the culture of the clinician can influence the interpretation of the patient's complaints and behaviors. Thus, there is a lot of room for cultural influence in the clinical assessment.

Mental health assessment is a dynamic process that involves multiple levels of interaction between the patient (and sometimes the patient's family) and the clinician (Tseng 1997; Tseng 2003). This dynamic process involves a series of steps. It starts with the distress or problems experienced and perceived by the patient, and proceeds to the presentation of complaints made by the patient to the clinician. These are perceived and understood as specific types of problems by the clinician, and finally an assessment of the disorder in question—which includes categorization and diagnosis—is made by the clinician. Thus, it is a process involving different steps or compartments. The following discussion elaborates this process in more detail.

Experience of Problems or Distress (by the Patient)

This refers to the distress the patient experiences inside of himself. A person experiences *pain* when he is hit; feels *anxious* if he is worried about something; becomes *paranoid* if he suspects that he is being persecuted by others; or has the feeling of going *downhill* if he has lost something significant to him. All these reactions to distress, which may be manifested as symptoms or signs, are subjective, experiential phenomena. These subjective reactions cannot be precisely measured from the outside. It is therefore impossible to know to what extent the actual *experience* of distress is influenced by cultural factors.

It is clear, however, that the forerunner of the distress—namely, the stress itself—can be impacted by sociocultural factors. Stress can be produced by culture in numerous ways. Stress can be produced by culturally demanded performance. For example, many cultures demand that a woman produce a male child; the society blames her, and the woman feels guilty, if she fails to bear a boy. Many societies expect children to achieve high academic performance; if the child fails to meet such parental expectations, he is shamed. Stress can be created by culturally maintained beliefs. For instance, if a person believes that it is very important to define the territory between sea and land, and he breaks a culturally held taboo and brings food across the land-sea territory, he may develop severe anxiety and associated somatic complaints—described as *Malgri* reaction (as observed in island people near Australia). If a person believes that it is fatal if his penis shrinks into his abdomen, he may become fearful that his penis is *shrinking* in response to such a cultural belief, and develop a panic response known as *koro*.

Perception of Problems or Disorders (by the Patient)

Following the experience of distress and the development of symptoms, the next step is for the patient to perceive and interpret the distressful experience that he is having. How he perceives and interprets it is a psychological phenomenon that is subject to the influence of cultural factors, in addition to other variables such as the patient's personality, knowledge, and psychological needs.

Based on how the problem is understood and perceived by the patient, the patient will show a secondary process of various reactions to the distress that he is experiencing. For instance, if a person interprets the chest pain he is having as nothing but chest pain, he will react to it relatively lightly. If he interprets it as the sign of an impending heart attack, however, he may become very anxious—even to the point of panic—further complicating the primary symptom of chest pain he is suffering. In a similar way, if a person believes that shrinking of the penis into the abdomen is fatal, he will react severely to any sign of possible penis shrinkage, even if the penis never shrinks into the abdomen (this syndrome has occurred in epidemics in Southeast Asia). If a person does not adhere to such beliefs, he will be impervious to normal changes to his body. In other words, the patient's perception of and reaction to the primary symptoms will add secondary symptoms that compound the clinical picture. The process of forming secondary symptoms is usually subject to cultural influences.

Presentation of Complaints or Illness (by the Patient or His or Her Family)

The next step is how the complaints or illness are presented by the patient to others—the process and art of *complaining* (this subject was covered in Chapter 4: Culture and Clinical Assessment). Analysis of this process has shown that how the problem, symptom, or illness is presented or communicated to the clinician will be based on the patient's (or his or her family's) orientation to illness, perceived meaning of the symptoms, motivation for help-seeking, and culturally expected or sanctioned *problem-presenting style*. It is a combination of the results of these factors that affects the process of complaining. But, there is definitely a clear role for culture to play in this complaining process. This is true for any medical problem, but particularly for mental disorders—or, as commonly occurs, when psychological issues are prominent in the medical condition.

For instance, patients of a given ethnic group may tend to make somatic complaints at their initial sessions with a mental health practitioner, despite being referred for psychological problems. There may be several alternative explanations of this rather common presentation. These include a physical condition is the patient's primary concern, somatic symptoms are being used as socially recognized signals of illness, somatic symptoms are a culturally sanctioned prelude to revealing psychological problems; or symptoms may be a reflection of hypochondriacal traits that are shared by the group (Tseng 1975). Thus, the nature of a presenting somatic complaint needs careful evaluation and understanding, rather than simply dealing with the somatic complaint itself or giving it the label of somatoform disorder.

In the reverse of this situation, a patient from another ethnic background may present many psychological problems to the therapist at the initial session, complaining that, as a small child, he was abused by some adult, was never adequately loved by his parents, and is now confused about his own identity, unclear about the meaning of life, and so on. It is necessary for the clinician to determine how much of this psychoanalyzed complaint may merely reflect the patient's learned behavior from public communication about patienthood, and how much of it is really his primary concern.

Perception and Understanding of the Disorder (by the Clinician)

A clinician, as a human being, a cultural person, and a professional, has his or her own ways of perceiving and understanding the complaints that are presented by patients. His or her psychological sensitivity, cultural awareness, professional orientation, and experience—as well as medical competence—will all act together to influence the assessment of the problems a patient has presented. The cultural background of the clinician is a significant factor, and deserves special attention, particularly when the clinician is examining a patient with a different cultural background—one with which the clinician is unfamiliar.

How the clinician's own cultural background affects the clinical assessment was shown in a study of the assessment of parent-child behavior by Japanese and American psychiatrists (Tseng et al. 1982). A series of videotaped family interaction patterns was shown to child psychiatrists in Tokyo and Honolulu, respectively. The clinicians of the two cultures reached remarkably different assessment conclusions. In one videotape, a father did not interact with his daughter, leaving this role to his wife. Japanese child psychiatrists tended to view this as exhibiting *adequate* and *all right* parenting behavior, while their American counterparts viewed such behavior as *not involved* and *inadequate* parenting behavior. The main reason for these different assessments was the clinicians' cultural expectations of a father's behavior. For Americans, it is culturally expected that the father, like the mother, should interact and be involved with all of his children, while the Japanese consider it more the mother's job to interact and be involved with the children, and not routinely an appropriate role for the father. If a father interacts directly and frequently with his daughter, it is considered *inappropriate behavior* in Japanese culture. This clearly demonstrates that a clinician's value system and cultural beliefs affect his way of making assessments.

It is well-recognized that the clinician's style of interviewing, perception of and sensitivity toward pathology, and familiarity with the disorder under examination all influence the interactions between patient and clinician—which, in turn, influence the outcome of the clinician's understanding of the disorder.

For example, an Asian patient's idiomatic complaints of suffering due to *weakness of the kidney* (a psychosexual problem), *elevated fire in the body or liver* (representing anger or anxiety), *loss of soul* (meaning feeling depressed or alienated), *disturbance from a deceased aunt's spirit*, and so on, may not be fully comprehended with cultural empathy by a Western clinician; while the problems of polysubstance abuse or psychosexual problems presented by a Western patient may be unfamiliar to an Asian clinician, who may be at a loss as to how to relevantly explore and understand the problem.

In sum, making a clinical assessment and diagnosis is a complex matter involving a dynamic process between the help-seeker and the help-provider. This assessment and diagnostic process is influenced in a variety of ways by the cultural background of the *patient*, as well as that of the *clinician*. The clinician should be aware of how cultural factors will affect each step in the process of interaction between the patient and the clinician.

The Ways in Which Culture Contributes to Psychopathology

In medical practice, there will occasionally be concerns how the specific pathology varies by ethnic group or race, but seldom are cultural factors considered to actually affect a specific disease. However, in mental healthcare, cultural factors can shape the psychopathology in several ways (Tseng & Streltzer 1997). They are pathoplastic effects, pathoselective effects, pathofacilitative effects, and pathogenic effects.

Pathoplastic Effects

This refers to the ways in which culture contributes to the appearance or molding of the manifestations of psychopathology. Culture shapes symptom manifestations at the level of the content presented. The content of delusions, auditory hallucinations, obsessions, or phobias is subject to the environmental context in which the pathology is manifested. For instance, an individual's grandiose delusions may be characterized by the belief that he is a Russian emperor, Jesus Christ, Buddha, the president of the United States, or the prime minister of the United Kingdom, depending on which figure is more popular or important in his society. If a person develops a delusional disorder with ideas of persecution, based on his social background the person who follows him, tries to poison him, or otherwise persecutes him, may be either a member of the CIA, the KGB, a communist, a political enemy, a deceased person's malicious spirit, an evil spirit, or an agent from outer space. Thus, the specific content of psychotic thinking is shaped by, and thus relevant to, the psychotic person's cultural background.

Pathoselective Effects

This refers to the tendency of some people in a society, when encountering stress, to select certain culturally influenced reaction patterns that result in the manifestation of certain psychopathologies. In Japan, for example, cultural influences lead a family encountering serious stress or a hopeless situation to choose, from among many alternative solutions, to commit suicide together—forming the unique psychopathology of *family suicide* observed in Japanese society. A Malaysian man humiliated in public, following cultural custom, is expected to take a weapon and kill people indiscriminately to show his manhood—an occurrence called an *amok* attack. Without their knowing it, culture has a powerful influence on the choices people make in reaction to stressful situations and shapes the nature of the psychopathology that occurs as a result of those choices. This only applies to minor (nonpsychotic) psychiatric disorders, particularly culture-related specific syndromes, not to major (psychotic) psychiatric disorders.

Pathofacilitative Effects

This implies that although cultural factors do not change the manifestation of the psychopathology too much—that is, the clinical picture can still be recognized and categorized without difficulty in the existing classification system—cultural factors do contribute significantly to the frequent occurrence of certain mental disorders in a society. In other words, the disorder potentially exists and is recognized globally, yet—due to cultural factors—it becomes prevalent in certain cultures at particular times. Thus, *facilitating* effects make it easier for certain psychopathologies to develop and increase their frequency. For instance, the excessive concern with body weight and the perception of slimness as beauty may facilitate the occurrence of excessive dieting and even a pathological eating disorder; a liberal attitude toward weapons control may result in more weapon-related violence or homicidal behavior; cultural permission to consume alcohol freely may increase the prevalence of drinking problems.

Pathogenic Effects

This refers to situations in which culture is a direct causative factor in forming or *generating* psychopathology. Cultural ideas and beliefs contribute to stress, which, in turn, produces psychopathology. Stress can be created by culturally formed anxiety, culturally demanded performance, and culturally prescribed restricted roles with special duties. Therefore, culture is considered to be a causative factor because culturally shared specific beliefs or ideas contribute *directly* to the formation of a particular stress—which, in turn, induces a certain mode of psychopathology. The psychopathology that occurs tends to be a culturally related specific syndrome—for instance, the folk belief that death will result if the penis shrinks into the abdomen, inducing the *koro* panic; or the popular anxiety over the *harmful* leaking of semen, leading to the development of the semen-loss anxiety disorder (or *dhat* syndrome).

Cultural Influences on Types of Psychopathology

It is important to recognize there are different ways or degrees in which culture impacts psychopathology, depending on the different types of disorders or the nature of psychopathology. Generally speaking, psychopathology that is predominantly determined by biological factors (such as organic mental disorders or psychoses) is less influenced by cultural factors, and any such influence is secondary or peripheral. In contrast, psychopathology that is predominantly determined by psychological factors (such as anxiety, depression, or other kinds of minor psychiatric disorders) is attributed more to cultural factors. This basic distinction is necessary in discussing different levels of cultural impact on various types of psychopathologies.

Depression

The cultural aspects of depression have created a keen interest among cultural psychiatrists since the 1960s. This interest coincided with the availability of antidepressants for treatment, but was motivated by the discovery that—in spite of a sharply increasing clinical trend of diagnosing depression in Euro-American societies—there seemed to be a low prevalence of it in non-Western societies.

To explain the possible reason for the low prevalence of depression diagnosed in non-Western societies, some clinicians used the concept of *masked depression* developed in the past. This concept takes the view that when certain individuals react to loss or frustration, instead of manifesting the emotional reaction of depression, they show other clinical pictures, such as somatic symptoms or behavior problems. This view is founded on the basic assumption that when a person encounters the psychological trauma of loss or frustration, he or she responds primarily with the mood disorder of *depression*. If, for some reason, the person is not able to respond with depression, and the trauma of loss or frustration is manifested by another mental condition, it is considered to be *masked* depression. This clinical assumption is misleading in cross-cultural applications. It assumes that human beings are allowed to react emotionally only in a defined way, ignoring that there are rich variations in the emotional and behavioral reactions of human beings in different cultural environments through patho-plastic effects. It is biased in identifying one reaction as primary and others as *masked*.

A recent study examined the association of pain complaints with mood and anxiety disorders—surveying over 85,000 subjects in 17 countries. The presence of multiple sites of pain symptoms were found to be strongly and consistently associated with such mental disorders in diverse cultures. The authors concluded that the concepts of pain representing culture-specific idioms of distress including masked depression were not justified (Gureje, Von Korff, Kola et al. 2007)

From a cultural perspective, it is more useful to understand the problem- presentation styles (or patterns) manifested by patients. As elaborated previously, the information and problems presented by patients to physicians are subject to various factors—including patient-therapist relations, culturally molded patterns of making complaints, and the clinical settings in which the interactions take place. This also applies to depression. Complaining about depression versus somatic symptoms deserves careful evaluation and consideration. Simon and colleagues (1999) used data from the World Health Organization (WHO) study of psychological problems in general healthcare to examine the relationship between somatic symptoms and depression. They found that among patients studied at 15 primary care centers in 14 countries on five continents around the world, about 10 percent who presented somatic symptoms to the primary caretaker met the criteria for major depression. Furthermore, they revealed that a somatic presentation was more common at medical centers where patients lacked an ongoing relationship with a primary care physician than at centers where most patients had a personal physician. This indirectly supports the view that the nature of complaints made by patients is closely related to patient-doctor relationships—namely, the patient will be more comfortable revealing personal matters and concern to their physician with whom they have long-time relationsships and are familiar with.

Recently, Bhui and his colleagues (2004) in the United Kingdom studied white European and Asian patients (who identified themselves as Punjabi originally from India) in general practices in southeast London. They reported that Punjabis had higher rates of depression than English subjects, with particularly high rates among women and those with physical disabilities. These findings contradict previous research showing lower rates of depression among South Asian primary care attendees. They stress that the dynamics of communication in the doctor-patient relationship, addressing how expression of somatic symptoms, and physical and psychological complaints will influence professional assessment.

Current evidence supports the contention that cultural variations in the prevalence of depressive disorders have to do with diagnostic trends rather than intrinsic differences. Non-Western presentations of symptoms are more likely to emphasize somatic presentations, and perhaps in a related way, are associated with different thresholds for assessing criteria for depression (Chang, Hahm, Lee, Shin, Jeon, Hong, Lee, Lee, & Cho 2007).

Cultural variations are recognized even among clinically recognized conditions of mood-related depression. In the late 1960s, German cultural psychiatrist Wolfgang Pfeiffer (1968) reviewed literature on depression in non-European cultures. He pointed out that the *core* symptoms of depression (i.e., change of mood, disruption of physiological functions, such as sleep and appetite, and hypochondriacal symptoms) in these cultures were the same as in Europe. However, other symptoms—such as feelings of guilt and suicidal tendencies—showed variations of frequency and intensity among cultures. This view was later supported by other investigators (Binitie 1975; Sartorius 1975).

For instance, based on clinical observation of depressive illnesses in Afghanistan, Waziri (1973) reported that the majority of depressed patients expressed *death wishes* instead of suicidal intentions or thoughts. In Afghanistan, people with Muslim backgrounds believe suicide is a sin. It is a cause of serious guilt to destroy the life that is given by God. Waziri said that the depressed patients who were asked how they viewed life answered that they "wished they were dead" or that they had "prayed to God to take their life away." Actually, the suicide rate among the general population was very low, namely 0.25 per 100,000 population (Gobar 1970), which was extremely low—the average rate for most countries is about 10 per 100,000 population per year. This illustrates that, even though a suicidal tendency is often associated with depression, cultural attitudes either sanctioning or forbidding self-destruction can modify the expression of suicidal ideas through a pathoplastic effect.

The presence or absence of self-deprecation—self-blame in the form of feeling ashamed or guilty—is another aspect that has gained attention and has been debated from cross-cultural perspectives. According to Prince (1968), mental-emotional self-castigation is rare or absent in the early stages of depressed patients in Africa,. Murphy, Wittkower and Chance (1967) have proposed that the higher incidence of guilt feelings in Western cultures was perhaps due to the influence of the Christian religion. However, after examining depressed Christian and Muslim patients in Cairo, Egypt, El-Islam (1969) reported that the presence or absence of guilt feelings was often associated with the level of education or literacy, and the degree of depression, rather than religious background. He concluded that guilt and Christianity are not necessarily closely linked for many people.

Clearly defined and sharply delineated depressive disorders are not typical in patient populations. Rather, the phenomenology is often mixed with anxiety and somatic presentations. This is true for patients from Western countries (such as the United States) and, even more so, from societies with different cultures. Depressive disorders include various clinical conditions on a spectrum that ranges from primarily biologically determined depressive *disorders* (exemplified by endogenous, periodically occurring depression) to predominantly psychologically related, context-based, depressive *reactions*. The human mind does not respond to an internal or external situation purely according to a defined *disorder*. This is particularly true when a person is reacting to psychological distress. The response is often a combination of anxiety, depression, anger, a feeling of frustration, and many concomitant physiological symptoms. This is particularly important for cross-cultural applications. Diagnostically mixed types of disorders are more the rule than the exception.

Anxiety and Related Disorders

If a patient manifests anxiety as a primary symptom, the diagnosis is usually at least one of the anxiety disorders. Many patients suffering from anxiety, instead of (or in addition to) complaining of anxiety, worries, or feelings of tenseness, present primarily with associated symptoms such as sleep disturbance, poor appetite, lethargy, headache, or irritability. Furthermore, depressive complaints can be prominent leading to a mixed picture of anxiety and depression.

In Japan, some patients manifest a unique type of anxiety—a social phobia characterized by symptoms of excessive self-consciousness, associated with a fear of flushing, concern with one's bodily orders, making gas, fear of eye-to-eye contact with others, fear of relating to intermediately-familiar persons (such classmates, or friends). In its severest form, there may be complete withdrawal from social activities (Yamashita 1977/1993). This condition is clinically regarded by Japanese clinicians as *taijinkyofushoo* (literally means fear of, or phobia about, interpersonal relations). It is said to be more prevalent in adolescents and young adults. In the past, it was regarded by Japanese psychiatrists as a culture-related specific syndrome observed in Japanese society, which is notable for its sensitive and delicate concerns about proper social relations (Kimura 1982). However, Korean psychiatrists recently reported that such a clinical condition is observed among Korean youth, as well (Lee 1987). A subtype of *taijinkyofushoo*, termed the *offensive* subtype, refers to a fear of behaving in a way that is socially inappropriate and offends others. Features of the offensive subtype of *taijinkyofushoo* have been found to be common among American patients with social anxiety disorder and may not be as culturally specific as previously believed (Choy, Schneier, Heimberg, Oh & Liebowitz (2007).

In Africa, the term *malignant anxiety* has been used by cultural psychiatrists (Lambo 1962) to address a unique clinical condition observed among some patients in which anxiety symptoms are accompanied by aggressive behavior toward others. This phenomenon occurs among young men who are frustrated by an inability to adjust to a rapidly changing society.

There are a number of disorders that are thought to be unique to specific cultures that are variants of anxiety disorders. These include *dhat* syndrome, *koro*, and *huabyong*, which are categorized as culture-related specific psychiatric syndromes and will be elaborated briefly later.

Somatization Disorders

If the patient complains primarily of somatic symptoms when there is no medical explanation, a somatoform disorder may be diagnosed consistent with the DSM classification system. If the patient is preoccupied with fears of having a serious medical disease based on a misinterpretation of bodily symptoms, it is categorized as hypochondriasis. From a cultural point of view, we can speculate that, in a society in which emotional expression is not encouraged but somatic complaints are more acceptable and facilitate attention from others, patients may tend to make somatic presentations even when psychological complaints would be more accurate. Somatoform disorders such as hypochondriasis will be more prevalently diagnosed (Tseng 1975; Kawanishi 1992).

The diagnostic term *neurasthenia* was originally coined in 1869 by the American neuropsychiatrist, George M. Beard, to describe a clinical syndrome with core symptoms of mental fatigue associated with poor memory, poor concentration, irritability, headaches, tinnitus, insomnia, and other vague somatic complaints. Beard believed that the disorder derived from an exhaustion of the victim's nervous system. The diagnostic term spread around the world, and it was referred to as *shenjin shuairuo* in China, and *shinkei shuijaku* in Japan—literally meaning *exhaustion of nerve*. Interestingly enough, since 1968 the term has been discarded from the formal classification system of DSM in America where the term was originated, reasoning that the clinical picture was not clearly defined, and weakness of the nervous system was misleading. However, the diagnostic term of neurasthenia is still prevalently used in China, Japan, and Korea and other countries, and the term is still retained in the international classification system, ICD-10.

Studying Chinese rural peasant patients, Chang and her colleagues (2005) reported that among the 49 subjects studied, 27 cases met the criteria for the current DSM-IV diagnoses of undifferentiated somatoform disorder (30.6 %), somatoform pain disorder (22.4%), somatization disorder (4.1%), or hypochondriasis (2%). The remaining 22 cases (44.9%), however, did not meet the criteria for any core DSM-IV diagnosis. They indicated that, rather than attempting to apply affective, anxiety, or somatoform disease constructs to these (neurasthenic) patients, there may be therapeutic benefits to retaining the diagnosis of *shenjin shuairuo* in the immediate future. As physicians, it is important to know that this term is used still by many Asian patients and clinicians.

Conversion and Dissociation Disorders

Among nonpsychotic psychiatric disorders, conversion and dissociation disorders are good examples of the rich effects of culture. The prevalence of conversion or dissociation varies greatly among different societies. It is also clear that in some societies—in contrast to other forms of psychopathology—it is preferable to deal with stress by repressing or dissociating painful emotion. Although some theories have been proposed to explain why certain cultural traits or certain child-rearing patterns favor the occurrence of conversion or dissociation, there is not yet any solid data to support such speculation. However, it is obvious that different societies have different reactions to the phenomena of conversion or dissociation, which, in turn, may facilitate the occurrence of the psychopathologies.

Culture-Related Specific Psychiatric Syndromes

Psychiatric syndromes that are significantly culture-related, with unique presentations that are recognized and labeled with folk terms by the local population, are not classifiable in the existing psychiatric classification system. These are addressed as culture-related specific psychiatric syndromes (or culture-bound syndromes). Although such syndromes are rare, and physicians seldom encounter such syndromes in usual clinical practice, it is useful to be aware of these unique and fascinating psychiatric syndromes and the folk terminology associated with them (Tseng 2003). Following are examples of some that are more or less related to physical conditions.

Koro (Genital-Retraction Anxiety Disorder)

Also referred to as *suoyang* (the term literally means *shrinkage of the penis*) in Chinese, this is a clinical condition in which the patient is morbidly concerned that his penis is shrinking or retracting—possibly to the point of disappearing—and dangerous consequences (such as death) might occur. Often observed among Chinese patients, it may occur as an epidemic involving many patients (Tseng 2001, Pp 217–224).

Naeng Syndrome (Leukorrhea Anxiety)

Naeng is the Korean word for leukorrhea. Leukorrhea is a whitish vaginal discharge that occurs normally, and varies with hormone cycles. Women complaining of *naeng* have been reported to frequent gynecological clinics in South Korea (Sich 1979). The patients are unusually insistent and persevering in wanting to eliminate this condition, and are not reassured when they are told that they have no clinical disorder causing the vaginal discharge. In spite of this, patients will exert great effort and spend a lot of money seeking treatment in different settings. At times, a hysterectomy has even been offered as a way to achieve relief from the discharge that the patients are concerned about, especially when minor anatomical changes are found, such as a Nabothian cyst and a medical diagnosis of *chronic cervicitis* is given to satisfy the patient.

One explanation for the behavior of these women can be found in the fact that the Korean word for leukorrhea—*naeng*—is synonymous with the word for *cold*. In Korean culture, and related to traditional Chinese medical concepts of yin and yang, the term *cold* implies an illness that is caused by the disruption of harmony between the opposite forces of yin and yang in the human body. Thus, to the Korean patients, *naeng* is a sign of an underlying *cold* condition, resulting in excessive discharge of a cold element.

Dhat Syndrome (Semen-Loss Anxiety)

Often seen among young male patients of India background, and based on the folk belief that semen is vital to health, the patient is very much concerned about the leaking of semen (Wig 1960; Neki 1973). Dhat syndrome is frequently associated with depressive symptoms. If DSM-IV criteria for major depression are met, antidepressant medication may be helpful (Dhikav, Aggarwal, Gupta, Jadhavi & Singh 2007).

Frigophobia (Morbid Fear of Catching Cold)

This disorder is seen mostly among Chinese patients. According to Chinese traditional theory of yin and yang, an imbalance between yin and yang will result in this disorder. It is based on the belief that excessive yin—caused by cold air or excessive eating of cold food—will result in weakness and sickness (Rin 1966; Chang et al. 1975).

Hwabyung (Fire Sickness)

Presented mostly by Korean women patients, this is a folk idiom of distress characterized by a wide range of somatic and emotional symptoms—including the feeling of pressure in the chest, pounding heart, and a fire sensation rising within the body or pain in the body. These clinical complaints usually occur when the patient encounters an intolerable emotional stress in the family setting (such as conflict with a mother-in-law). It has been interpreted that the patient is suffering from accumulated resentment (Lee 1977).

Susto (Soul Loss)

This is a Spanish word that literally means *fright*. The term is widely used by people in Latin America to refer to a loss of soul. It is based on the folk belief that if a person loses his soul due to being frightened or startled, he will manifest certain morbid mental conditions, and will need to recapture the soul by performing healing rituals (Rubel 1964).

Schizophrenia

Schizophrenia is a commonly occurring major psychiatric disorder. It has been studied intensely from biological, psychological, social, and cultural perspectives.

Since the late 1970s, the World Health Organization has carried out several investigations concerning schizophrenia. It was found that the incidence rates did not differ much among the various countries studied—ranging from 0.7 to 1.4 per 10,000 population aged 15 to 54. (Jablensky et al. 1991, pp 45–52). The similar incidence among countries with different cultures supports the notion that schizophrenia tends to occur predominantly due to biological-hereditary factors. There is only a pathoplastic effect on the manifestations of the symptomatology, including the subtypes of schizophrenia.

Substance Abuse and Dependency

Mental disorders associated with substance abuse and/or dependency are basically biophysiological in nature, however there is room for psychological influence. Culture has patho-selective and patho-facilitative effects on the prevalence of abuse. For instance, if a society takes a firm attitude against drinking, such as most Muslim societies, alcohol consumption is very low and problems associated with alcohol are relatively rare. In contrast, if a society takes a relatively liberal attitude toward drinking, such as most Euro-American societies and the Asian societies of Korea and Japan, alcohol consumption is very high and the prevalence of alcohol-related problems is similarly higher. Indulgence in alcohol and other intoxicating substances become culturally available—even favored choices—as a way of dealing with stress.

The risk of alcohol and substance abuse disorders greatly increases when there is rapid socio-cultural change, particularly associated with cultural uprooting—substance abuse tends to increase sharply. For many culturally deprived minority groups, the problems of substance abuse and dependency, particularly among young people, are substantial and serious.

Suicidal Behavior

Suicide is a multidimensional clinical phenomenon. Suicidal behavior is usually seen as a complication of psychiatric disorders, usually associated with depression or irrational thought. It is often associated with substance abuse or dependence. However, suicidal behavior varies widely by country, and may reflect the distress that exists in a society or cultural system.

Based on data available from the World Health Organization, supplemented by resources from individual investigators, several findings stand out (Tseng 2001,

Table 22-1). There is a rather wide range of rates among the different countries. The *very high* group consists of countries with total suicide rates above 25 per 100,000 population. Hungary, Sri Lanka, Micronesia, Finland, and Austria belong to this group. The *high* group has total suicide rates between 15 and 25 per 100,000 population. South Korea, Japan, Switzerland, Denmark, and Germany belong to this group. Many countries, including the United States, France, the United Kingdom, Belgium, and Canada, belong to the *moderate* group, which has total suicide rates between 10 and 15 per 100,000 population. The *low* group, with total suicide rates between 5 and 10 per 100,000 population, includes New Zealand, Norway, the Netherlands, and Italy. Several countries, such as Mexico, Egypt, Malaysia, and the Philippines—with total suicide rates below 5 per 100,000 population—belong to the *very low* group. Many of the *very low* rate countries are Muslim or Catholic societies that have prohibitive religious attitudes toward self-killing.

In addition to the difference in suicide rates among different cultures, it is important to know that from aclinical point of view the presentation of suicidal ideas are tremendously subject to cultural factors. Revealing the presence of suicidal thoughts may be more strongly avoided by people from certain cultures, such as those strongly influenced by Islam or Catholicism, because self-injury or self-induced death is not accepted by their religious community. For people in other cultures—even those with higher suicide rates (such as in Asia)—it may be considered shameful to indicate that they have suicidal thoughts. This is particularly true for men in cultures where the idealized man exhibits strength and courage. Thoughts of suicide may appear to be a sign of weakness. Thus, there needs to be special consideration and effort during the clinical assessment of suicidality because it may not be culturally easy for such a patient to reveal suicidal impulses. On the other hand, in some societies (such as America), suicidal ideation is an effective means to get attention from physicians, and such complaints may be offered (particularly among homeless people) by patients who desire to be hospitalized for food, shelter, or to avoid having to care for themselves.

Mental Disorders Associated with Brain Dysfunction

By definition, these brain disorders are caused by organic etiological factors. Thus, culture does not have a *direct* causal effect on these conditions. Also, the phenomenology of disorders caused by specific brain pathologies will be relatively similar, - regardless of the ethnic or cultural background of the patient. However, cultural factors—such as a unique lifestyle collectively shared by a group of people—may *indirectly* contribute to the occurrence, or influence the prevalence, of certain organic mental disorders.

A good example is the degenerative disease of the nervous system called *kuru* among the Fore tribe people of New Guinea. For years (until recently), about 1 percent of the population (mainly women) would die annually from this fatal disease. The Fore people themselves believed that *kuru* was caused by sorcery. One of the great discoveries of contemporary medicine was the finding that *kuru* is a disease caused by a virus that attacks the central nervous system after a long incubation period (Harter 1974). It was the custom for Fore women to ritually eat the bodies and brains of their relatives when they died (Keesing 1976), thus consuming the virus, which allowed the disease to be transmitted through the females. This illustrates clearly that, while culture does not cause this organic disease of the central nervous system, the culture-rooted habit of eating human brains contributes significantly, though secondarily, to the transmission of the organic mental disorder.

Another example is sexual behavior related to organic mental disorders, such as neurosyphilis, gonoencephalitis, or AIDS-related neuropsychopathy. While culture is not an etiological factor in these organic mental disorders, a society's attitude toward sexual behavior—particularly outside of marriage—and its tolerance of promiscuity will certainly affect the sexual behavior of its members. This, in turn, will influence the prevalence of sexually transmitted diseases and resulting mental complications.

Personality Disorders

Different cultures emphasize different personality traits as ideal. Therefore, defining or labeling deviations from *normal personality* is a culture-relative exercise, whose boundaries are reflective of the specific values, ideas, worldview, resources, and social structure of the society (Foulks 1996). For instance, dependent personality disorder is defined as "having difficulty making everyday decisions without an excessive amount of advice and reassurance from *others*," and "needing *others* to assume responsibility for most major areas of his or her life." This definition needs careful consideration, depending on whether the person concerned is living in an individual or a collective society. In a collective society, consideration of, consulting with, and allowing or even depending on others to lead and help is a cultural expectation that does not necessarily imply that the person is suffering from a dependent personality.

The concept of antisocial personality disorder is defined by the failure to conform to *social norms*, having problems maintaining culturally desirable interpersonal social relations (such as reckless disregard for the safety of others, deceitfulness, or aggressiveness), and a lack of socially expected guilty feelings for wrongful behavior. Some cultures, however, are more likely to accept and sometimes admire behavior that is rebellious and even challenges authority. Antisocial personality disorders are more likely to flourish in such societies. These societies are more likely to be part of Western cultures. Clearly, socio-cultural judgment in particular is needed to define those personality disorders.

Psychopharmacological Therapy

Many psychiatric disorders can be treated rather successfully by medication, and drug therapy should be considered whenever it is indicated. However, from racial and cultural points of view, there are three issues deserving attention.

The first one is the possible racial influence on psychopharmacological therapy. Although there is a lot of overlap, there are differences in pharmacodynamic and pharmacokinetic effects of many medications for different racial groups. Generally speaking, the dose for medication needs to be less for certain racial or ethnic groups. For instance, doses for psychotropic medications are recommended to be two-thirds or less for patients with Asian ancestry than those recommended for patients with European-American ancestry. This is recommended both in terms of the dose needed for effectiveness, and to minimize side effects. Needless to say, there are individual variations within each racial or ethnic group, so clinical judgment is required and one cannot rely on a hard and fast rule (Lin et al. 1993; Lin et al. 1995).

The second issue is regarding nongenetic biological factors. Medication can be greatly influenced by many biological factors such as diet, drinking, or smoking habits. Simultaneous use of herbs for medicinal effects is another issue that deserves careful attention, because there is a considerable possibility of interaction between pharmaceutical medicines and herbal medicines.

The third issue concerns the psychology of prescribing and receiving medication (Ahmed 2001). Medicines facilitate particular social and symbolic processes (see Chapter 7). This includes the form or consistency of the drug, the sensory experience when the medication is taken, the source of the medicine, its packaging, and even the mode of administration. In general, injectable agents are believed to be more powerful than oral, for example. Finally, culture influences the nature of the doctor-patient relationship and the symbolic meaning of the transaction itself for all parties involved.

Psychological Therapy

Psychotherapy remains the mainstay of treatment for mental disorders. Clinical studies have indicated that—even for those disorders most responsive to medication, such as the psychoses—patient outcomes are better when combined with psychotherapy. Of course, many psychological conditions respond to medication no better than to placebos, and only psychotherapy can be considered efficacious.

From a cultural point of view, however, many patients whose background renders them unfamiliar with the practice of psychotherapy will be not able to recognize the importance of *talk therapy*. These patients need to be educated in a supportive way to understand the potential benefits of talking confidentially about their emotional problems. Once they get oriented to the therapeutic aspect of psychotherapy, they will make good use of it.

Of course, psychotherapy needs to be performed in a culturally competent manner that fits the patient's cultural background. At the same time, the therapist must evaluate his or her own culture and value system, because it can significantly affect the process, direction, and goals of the psychotherapy (Tseng & Streltzer 2001).

References

Ahmed I (2001) Psychological aspects of giving and receiving medications. In: Tseng WS Streltzer J (eds) Culture and psychotherapy: A guide to clinical practice. American Psychiatric Press, Washington D.C., pp123–134

Bhui K, Bhugra D, Goldberg D, Suer J, Tylee A (2004) Assessing the prevalence of depression in Punjabi and English primary care attenders: The role of culture, physical illness and somatic symptoms. Transcultural Psychiatry 41:307–322

Binitie A (1975) A factor-analytical study of depression across cultures (African and European). British Journal of Psychiatry 127:559–563

Chang DF, Myers HF, Yeung A, Zhang YL, Zhao JP, Yu SY (2005) *Shenjing shuairuo* and the DSM-IV: Diagnosis, distress, and disability in a Chinese primary care setting. Transcultural Psychiatric Research Review 42:204–218

Chang SM, Hahm BJ, Lee JY, Shin MS, Jeon HJ, Hong JP, Lee HB, Lee DW, Cho MJ (2007) Cross-national difference in the prevalence of depression caused by the diagnostic threshold. Journal of Affective Disorders. Aug 27 [Epub ahead of print]

Chang YH, Rin H Chen CC (1975) Frigophobia: A report of five cases. Bulletin Chinese Society of Neurology and Psychiatry 1(2):9–13 [in Chinese]

Choy Y, Schneier FR, Heimberg RG, Oh KS, Liebowitz MR (2007) Features of the offensive subtype of Taijin-Kyofu-Sho in US and Korean patients with DSM-IV social anxiety disorder. Depression and Anxiety. Mar 5 [Epub ahead of print]

Dhikav V, Aggarwal N, Gupta S, Jadhavi R Singh K (2007) Depression in Dhat Syndrome. Journal of Sexual Medicine. Apr 19 [Epub ahead of print]

El-Islam MF (1969) Depression and guilt: A study at an Arab psychiatric clinic. Social Psychiatry 4:56–58

Foulk EF (1996) Culture and personality disorders. In: Mezzich JE, Kleinman A, Fabrega H, Jr, Paron DI (eds) Culture and psychiatric diagnosis: A DSM-IV Perspectives. American Psychiatric Press, Washington D.C., pp 243–252

Gobar AH (1970) Suicide in Afghanistan. British Journal of Psychiatry 116:493–496

Gureje O, Von Korff M, Kola L, Demyttenaere K, He Y, Posada-Villa J, Lepine JP, Angermeyer MC, Levinson D, de Girolamo G, Iwata N, Karam A, Luiz Guimaraes Borges G, de Graaf R, Browne MO, Stein DJ, Haro JM, Bromet EJ, Kessler RC, Alonso J (2007) The relation between multiple pains and mental disorders: Results from the World Mental Health Surveys. Pain Jun 12. [Epub ahead of print]

Jablensky A, Sartorius N, Ernberg G, Anker M, Korten A, Cooper JE, Day R, Bertelsen A (1991) Schizophrenia: Manifestations, incidence and course in different cultures—A World Health Organization Ten-Country Study. Psychological Medicine, Monograph Supplement 20 Cambridge University Press, Cambridge

Kawanish Y (1992) Somatization of Asians: An artifact of Western medicalization? Transcultural Psychiatric Research Review 29:5–36

Kessing RM (1976) Cultural anthropology: A contemporary perspective. Hold, Rinehart & Winston New York, p 219

Kimura S (1982) Nihonjin no taijinkyofusho (Japanese anthrophobia) Tokyo: Keso Shobo. [in Japanese]

Lambo TA (1962) Malignant anxiety: a syndrome associated with criminal conduct in Africans. Journal of Mental Science 108:256–264

Lee SH (1977) A study on the "*hwabyung*" (anger syndrome). Journal of the Korean General Hospital 1:63–69

Lee SH (1987) Social phobia in Korea. In: Social Phobia in Japan and Korea—Proceedings of the First Cultural Psychiatry Symposium between Japan and Korea. The East Asian Academy of Cultural Psychiatry, Seoul

Lin KM, Poland RE, Anderson D (1995) Psychopharmacology, ethnicity, and culture. Transcultural Psychiatric Research Review 28:3–37

Lin KM, Poland RE, Nakasaki G (eds) (1993) Psychopharmacology and psychobiology of ethnicity. American psychiatric Press, Washington, D.C.

Murphy HBM, Wittkower ED, Chance N (1967) Crosscultural inquiry into the symptomatology of depression: A prelimianry report. International Journal of Psychiatry 3(1):6–22

Neki JS (1973) Psychiatry in South-east Asia. British Journal of Psychiatry 123:256–269

Offer D, Sabshin M (1974) Normality: Theoretical and clinical concepts of mental Health, 2nd edn. Basic Books, New York

Pfeiffer W (1968) The symptomatology of depression viewed transculturally. Transcultural Psychiatric Research Review 5:121–124

Prince R (1968) The changing picture of depressive syndromes in Africa: Is it fact or diagnostic fashion? Canadian Journal of African Studies 1:177–192

Rin H (1966) Two forms of vital deficiency syndrome among Chinese male mental patients. Transcultural Psychiatric Research Review 3:19–21

Rubel AJ (1964) The epidemiology of a folk illness: *Susto* in Hispanic America. Ethology 3:268–283

Sartorius N (1975) Epidemiology of depression. WHO Chronicle 29:423–427

Simon GE, VonKorff M, Piccinelli M, Fullerton C, Ormel J (1999) An international study of the relation between somatic symptoms and depression. New England Journal of Medicine 341(18):1329–1335

Tseng WS (1975) The nature of somatic complaints among psychiatric patients: The Chinese case. Comprehensive Psychiatry 16:237–245

Tseng WS (2001) Handbook of cultural psychiatry. Academic Press, San Diego

Tseng, WS (2003) Clinician's guide to cultural psychiatry Academic Press, San Diego

Tseng WS, McDermott JF Jr, Ogino K, Ebata K (1982) Cross-cultural differences in parent-child assessment: USA and Japan. International Journal of Social Psychiatry 28:305–317

Tseng WS, Streltzer J (eds) (1997) Culture and Psychopathology: A Guide to Clinical Assessment. Brunner/Mazel, New York

Tseng WS, Streltzer J (eds) (2001) Culture and Psychotherapy: A Guide to Clinical Practice. American Psychiatric Press, Washington D.C.

Waziri R (1973) Symptomatology of depressive illness in Afghanistan. American Journal of Psychiatry 130:213–217

Wig NN (1960) Problem of mental health in India. Journal of Clinical and Social Psychiatry, College of Lucknow, India 17 (2):48–53

Yamashita I (1993) Taijinkyofu or delusional social phobia. Hokkaido University Press, Sapporo (English translation of Japanese book originally published in 1977. Kanehara, Tokyo). Reviewed in Transcultural Psychiatry Research Review, 2:283–288 (1984)

Chapter 7
Culture and Medical Care

Most practitioners of medicine encounter patients of diverse ethnic and cultural backgrounds. Even having knowledge of and experience with cultural differences, cultural factors add to the challenge of medical practice.

Outpatient Care

In the United States, patients typically need to make appointments by phone before visiting physicians on an outpatient basis. Patients are not supposed to just drop in, as they can in hospital emergency departments. However, this is not necessarily true for people living in traditional or developing societies, where people just show up to see the local healer or physician. There are many practical reasons that these patients may not be able to make appointments ahead of time and keep a set schedule. There is often no access to phone, and transportation may be very limited. Public buses do not necessarily run on schedule. These factors, even if no longer present, have contributed to certain habits and expectations. People do not think that patients need to visit a doctor on time using an appointment system. Therefore, particularly for health clinics that provide service to patients with traditional backgrounds, the clinic serves best by preparing to receive the patient who arrives without an appointment.

Family Physician System

In contemporary medical practice, primary care physicians expect to continuously take care of their patients' medical needs, coordinating care with specialists as appropriate. Some patients, however, are not aware of this aspect of *medical culture*, and they see no problem in going to different doctors at different times—after advice from friends or family, and even after being influenced by rumors or advertisements. Several doctors or healers may be seen at the same time, including practitioners of alternative medicine or folk medicine. The primary care physician will do well to inquire about additional treatments that the patient has sought, and additional medications the patient may be taking.

Cultural Aspects of Hospitalization

Hospital Admission

The act of hospitalization itself has different psychological implications for each patient. Some people appreciate hospitalization as a necessary consequence of the need for intensive medical care, allowing them to receive adequate attention. Others become more preoccupied with the personal restrictions and loss of personal and family life that occurs in this medical setting.

The Experience of Hospitalization

Giger and Davihizar (1999, p 60) described the case of a man who reacted to the hospital setting. A 56-year old German immigrant, employed as an engineer, was admitted to the coronary care unit with chest pain and shortness of breath. The wife visited the patient, bringing personal items, including family portraits, roses from their home garden, and clothing. However, because the coronary care unit was restricted in space, personal items were not allowed, and the wife was instructed to take the items home. After two days, when the patient's symptoms subsided, he was transferred to a semiprivate room in the coronary care step-down unit, but with orders to remain on bed rest. The nurses observed that the patient was anxious, somewhat withdrawn, and unable to express his needs and feelings. The patient's emotional reaction to the hospitalization was interpreted as culturally based. The patient was used to being active and independent. He also was deprived of the family atmosphere that his wife attempted to recreate before the personal items were taken away. Culturally, some German people desire a larger space and are less flexible in their spatial behavior than some Americans. Germans often live in the same house their entire lives, whereas Americans change locations approximately every five years, and may be more content with temporary territories rather than permanent ones.

Many Micronesian or Polynesian patients have difficulty adjusting to the modern hospital. In their tropical island homes, they may have lived in a large hut house, open to the outside, without walls separating rooms inside the house. Many family members or relatives live together in the same open area, never feeling isolated. A small, air-conditioned patient room in a modern hospital is quite a contrast. The most uncomfortable part is not being surrounded by family members all the time.

For patients from Bali, Indonesia, the physical orientation of the bed is very important. Traditionally, these people believe that almighty God inhabits the mountain where the volcano erupts, and they customarily sleep with their head directed toward the north, where the volcano mountain is located. When admitted to a local hospital, built by Westerners without this consideration, the patients cannot sleep in comfort, because the beds were not arranged in the rooms to face north.

Medical Rules and Restrictions

Hospitalization does not simply mean coming to the hospital for intensive medical care—it also forces the patient to live in an artificial (medical) setting vastly different from their natural home setting. In addition to the psychological meanings of being admitted to the hospital, the admission deprives the patient of his or her personal lifestyle, and bends the norm of cultural patterns, resulting in many restrictions and impositions forced upon him or her by hospital regulations and the prevailing medical culture. These rules and restrictions deprive patients of the lifestyle they are used to having at home, requiring adjustments. There is distinctively different lifestyle at home and in the hospital—a remarkable cultural gap.

A Patient's Uniform

Modern hospitals require patients to wear hospital gowns. This makes it convenient for healthcare providers to identify patients, and to provide medical care easily, including physical examinations. Laundry is easily taken care of collectively. Hospital gowns also signify to patients that they have to act like patients—lying on the bed, following orders, and observing certain restrictions. For some patients, this may feel unnatural, depriving them of their individuality. Certain Micronesian patients may not be used to wearing shirts that cover the upper body, some Muslim women may feel the need to cover their hair, and the Japanese elderly may be uncomfortable not wearing *kimono* (traditional Japanese clothing). Should modern hospitals be concerned with these cultural issues? It deserves our attention.

Physicians' Rounds

For the sake of their own convenience (not that of patients), physicians customarily perform rounds at certain hours. Patients will generally have the opportunity to contact their attending physician directly only at such limited times. Surgeons usually make rounds early in the morning before scheduled operations. Thus, surgical patients must wake up very early to be able to talk to their surgeon. After rounds, internists and pediatricians may leave to see outpatients. The in-house patients will be seen only by nursing staff for the rest of the day unless there arises some urgent situation requiring the physician to visit again. The patient has no alternative but to accept and follow this part of medical culture. For some patients, this may be a difficult adjustment.

Informing the Patient and Family of the Diagnosis

An important part of medical practice is the physician's explanation of the disease in ways that the patient can understand and learn how to deal with it. Contemporary American healthcare professionals uphold a model of direct, truthful communication and information-sharing with patients. Physicians are encouraged to inform the patient of the actual diagnosis, even if the disease is a serious one. This is based on the belief that it is desirable for an individual (the patient) to take responsibility for medical decisions relating to his or her life. Currently, disclosure of medical information to patients is necessary because of the legal need to obtain the patient's informed consent to treatment, and is thus reinforced by concerns about malpractice suits.

From a psychological point of view, if the physician is not able to give a precise diagnosis of the diseases from which the patient is suffering, and comes across as vague, anxiety may develop in the patient as well as the family. Face the unknown or uncertainty provokes anxiety. This is true for any situation in which a person has serious problems, and may be even particularly so when a person is suffering from medical disorders. Although many patients cope by using denial in the face of medical distress, others are eager to know what is causing their condition and how to treat it.

However, in reality and from a medical point of view, a physician is not always able to make a firm diagnosis. Many medical conditions can be given only a speculative diagnosis. A physician naturally hesitates to prematurely give a firm diagnosis, to avoid the possibility of being incorrect if the diagnosis needs to be changed later. However, from psychological and cultural points of view, this may create doubt and mistrust on the part of the patient (or the family). People expect that, if the healer is competent, he or she will know the diagnosis and method of treatment right away. Within that cultural context, the healthcare professional that does not express confidence in a precise diagnosis may be seen as incompetent. This creates a dilemma: how to inform the patient (and family) about the diagnosis as precisely as possible, thereby instilling trust while also avoiding an incorrect or incomplete diagnosis.

Communicating the diagnosis to the patient and family requires professional skill to be accurate and realistic, yet maintain hope and sustain the ability to help the patient cope. Two areas deserve to be considered in this regard. One is patient's ability to understand the medical diagnosis, including the etiology and the principles of treatment. The patient's intelligence, educational level, and ability to comprehend the language (if the patient is not fluent in the language used by the physician or health professional) affect the patient's ability to understand. The other is the meaning or association attached to particular medical diseases for the patient. Based on social and cultural backgrounds, the patient may have sensitivities regarding certain diseases, especially ones with social stigma or false theories held by folk healers from the past. Laymen particularly fear certain medical disorders. Because venereal diseases are usually associated with socially unsanctioned sexual behavior, such as prostitution or promiscuity, such diseases are considered shameful in many societies and patients try to conceal them from others (see Chapter 5).

Krauses-Mars and Lachman (1994) studied the ethnic differences in South African parents' reactions to unfavorable news about their children. The parents of white and black preschool children with disabling medical diseases were asked about the explanations provided to them about the illnesses of their children. White parents—despite reporting that explanations were given by physicians—tended to deny the diagnosis of a mental illness more than other groups. Few black parents reported being asked about their understanding of the diagnosis. The investigators pointed out that the use of a language other than the patient's native tongue had a negative influence on communication between physician and parents. However, because the majority of the physicians are white in South Africa, racial attitudes held by physicians as well as patients' cultural attitudes toward unfavorable sicknesses might all have contributed to the process of explanation of disease between physicians and patients.

Disclosure of Bad News *about Terminal Illness*

In many cultures, there is substantial reluctance on the part of physicians and families to share correct diagnoses with the patient, particularly of the terminal illness. Contemporary American healthcare professionals believe that honest communication and information-sharing with dying patients is important, and physicians are encouraged to inform the patient of the actual diagnosis, even if the disease is a terminal one. This is based on the belief that it is desirable for a patient to take responsibility for medical decisions relating to his or her life. It is tempting to interpret this medical practice as a reflection of American values. Not that long ago, however, the great majority of American physicians believed that it was clinically best not to inform patients of a terminal illness (Oken 1961). The change in physicians' beliefs about this issue occurred in the 1960s and 1970s (Novack, Plumer, Smith, Ochitill, Morrow & Bennett 1979), reflecting a shift in the attitudes of the greater society toward authority during this period of cultural turmoil.

Beyene (1992) points out that for Ethiopians, *bad news* should be told to a close family member or friend of the patient who will divulge the information in a culturally approved time and manner. In the Arabic East, direct mention of death is avoided. In facing a fatal illness, patients, families, and physicians resort to elaborate forms of denial (Racy 1969). In Japan, the custom of keeping bad news from the patient is based on concerns that it may provoke suicidal ideas. The physician follows the family's wishes and tells the patient he has a less serious illness. If the physician were to inform the patient frankly about his terminal illness, the family may be upset at the *inconsiderateness* of the physician. Tang, Bultz, Zhang, and de Groot (2006) indicated that Asian cultures emphasize providing security, serenity, tranquility, and hope. The principle of nonmaleficence is the main reason for non-disclosure of bad news to patients. Folk people traditionally hold the view that a person is entitled to be treated as a *child* when ill, needing protection from worry and psychological burden. Culturally, it is beneficial to the patient's well-being to withhold painful information and thus, family members have honorable intentions in supporting nondisclosure of terminal illness to the patient. In Asian society, informing cancer patients about the disease and prognosis means giving a death sentence or a condemnation that can close possibilities and destroy hope. However, such traditional views are changing. In contemporary China, about three-quarters of people with cancer who are surveyed preferred to be informed of their cancer diagnosis, while one-quarter suggested that it would depend on their personal situation, and about 3 percent thought they should not be told (Tang, Bultz, Zhang, & de Groot 2006). A study in Hong Kong (Tse, Cong, & Fok 2003) revealed that 95 percent of people wanted information disclosed to them even if the news were bad. On the contrary, however, a recent study from Iran found that patients with gastrointestinal cancer who knew their diagnosis had a much higher rate of psychological distress than a control group of cancer patients who were unaware of their diagnosis (Tavoli, Mohagheghi, Montazeri, Roshan, Tavoli & Omidvari 2007).

Clearly, there exist widely different cultural views as to whether the physician should truthfully inform the patient about the diagnosis of a fatal disease. In some settings, it has been safest for the healthcare provider to discuss the matter with family first, and informing the patient has worked best with family members' understanding (or approval).

Consent for Medical Examination and Treatment

Implication of Making Consent

The legally oriented American society requires patients (and/or family) to give consent for examinations, tests, and treatment. They are asked to sign a written form so that it will be documented. This is relatively easy for patients or their family if, in their ordinary life, they are used to signing such documents—particularly in contemporary society that emphasizes law and values proper legal procedure. However, it may be puzzling or even frightening to those who are from other societies where the people rely on verbal communication and explanation and are not accustomed to signing formal documents. Extra effort may be needed to explain such to them.

Understanding Medical Authorization Documents

To sign a document is one thing, but to understand the content of the document that a patient is asked to sign is another matter. If the patient is not able to read the document, or is dependent on an interpreter, he or she may be confused, have misunderstandings, and even develop suspiciousness. Proper translation and suitable interpretation is needed. To compound the issue, such documents are often written in a formal (and legal) way that is not easily comprehended by laymen even if they can read the document.

Prescribing and Taking Medication

Patients' Beliefs and Attitudes toward Medication

Besides the medical and pharmacological aspects of medications, psychological issues influence the reaction to being prescribed drugs, the effectiveness of such prescription (e.g., adherence, the placebo effect), and the doctor-patient relationship. Culture, of course, has a major impact on these psychological influences.

Physical characteristics of medications, including color, size, and material, may have a psychological impact on the patient. The mode of administration of medicine has an impact as well (Ahmed 2001). Information that the patient has received from family, friends, or the popular media can also have a significant influence on a patient's reaction to medication and its effectiveness.

Western medicine is based on a pharmacotechnology that prepares a drug in a pure form to perform specific pharmacological functions. Modern physicians usually prescribe a single medication for a specific purpose, and for multiple problems they may prescribe multiple medications. Fewer medications are prescribed, if possible, to avoid drug interactions. In contrast, herbal medicine used in traditional medical practice is thought to work by combining multiple remedies in their raw form. Multiple herbs are always prescribed, as there is not too much concern over the use of compound medications. In societies where traditional medicine is still used, Western medicine is generally considered *strong* and useful for combating the specific etiology of a disorder, but there are usually unwelcome side effects. Traditional herbal medicine is viewed as *harmonious*, with fewer side effects, and will *strengthen* the body so that it can overcome the disorder. Herbal medicines may also have many (unnoticed) side effects, however, and are sometimes harmful to health.

A patient may have different preferences toward medication, not by its pharmacological effectiveness or undesirable side effects, but by the mode of prescription, appearance, color, and size of the pill that they are prescribed to take. Buckalew and Coffield (1982) discovered that the color of capsules affects placebo response differentially in different ethnic groups. For instance, white capsules were viewed by

Caucasian-Americans as analgesics and by African-Americans as stimulants in contrast to black capsules, which were viewed by Caucasian-Americans as stimulants and by African-Americans as analgesics. Furthermore, whether the medicine is derived from plants, animals, or is of synthetic origin can have a psychological impact on the medication response (Ahmed 2001, p 128). For instance, because of religious proscriptions, Muslims may not use alcohol-containing liquid medications. Muslims and orthodox Jews may not use medications containing porcine products. Vegetarians may not be willing to take medications with animal products in them.

Furthermore, it is important for healthcare providers to be aware that patients from certain cultural backgrounds may feel that there is no need to follow the physician's order in taking the medication. If the medicine works immediately (within a day or so), the patient will take the medication for a while. If the symptoms subside, the patient may decide to discontinue the medication even against the physician's directions. Kandakai, Price, Telljiohann, and Holiday-Goodman (1996) examined the use of antibiotics among African-Americans based on gender. Women were more likely to report completing the prescribed trial of antibiotics, while older men were more likely to use antibiotics only until the problem stopped. A significant percentage of men (23%) and women (18%) reported sharing their antibiotics with another person. Physicians should be aware of the patterns of compliance with medication, not only at the individual level but also at the ethnic/cultural level.

Case Example

A public health nurse visited an elderly Hawaiian patient to see how he was doing in the home setting. She was surprised to find that the patient kept more than 30 kinds of drugs in his medicine cabinet. Most had been prescribed several years before, and the expiration date had passed. The patient's wife informed the nurse that her husband often showed his medicine cabinet to his friends when they visited him, impressing upon them that he was not a well man. Furthermore, he would occasionally take a pill, choosing it based on color and taste. Also, he would offer the medicine to his relatives at times, if he felt they could benefit somehow by one or another of them.

Physicians' Patterns of Prescribing Medication

Patterns of prescribing medication are often affected by the psychology and culture of the physician beyond purely scientific reasons. Prescribing drugs to patients makes physicians feel that a *therapeutic* measure has been completed. Some physicians will rely primarily on medication or intervention management, while others use advice and support more freely. The different patterns of prescribing medication are clearly seen in the specialty of psychiatry. Some psychologically-minded psychiatrists will do psychological counseling more and prescribe medication less, while biologically-oriented psychiatrists tend to do the opposite—even for the same condition. In India, psychiatrists prescribe more drugs than in other societies, due to cultural issues regarding the status of psychiatry as a field of medicine (Nunley 1996).

Modern Western physicians make no secret about the name and nature of prescriptions, and often make it a goal to explain to the patient the drug's mechanism as well as potential side effects. Traditional physicians, on the other hand, sometimes keep prescriptions secret, and in some Asian countries such as Japan, China, and Korea, the patient may not expect the physician to give a full explanation.

In the United States, it is expected that the patient will be warned about the possible undesirable side effects of medications. It is sometimes thought necessary to list all the possible side effects so that the consent will be legally protected. However, it may frighten the patient (or family) to be aware of such terrible side effects. This increases the doubt and promotes noncompliance for taking the medication as prescribed. There is a clash between medical (and legal) culture and the patient's psychological needs. Explaining the possible undesirable side effects, but not scaring off the patient from taking the prescription, is a challenge that tests clinical skill.

Family Involvement in Medical Care

Although modern medicine recognizes the importance of involving family in the healthcare of the patient, this often does not occur for various reasons in practice. In the hospital setting (particularly intensive care), staff are concerned with the family's interference with the medical (often high-tech) needs of the patient. Staying away may be quite difficult for families of certain cultural backgrounds, such as Asian, Latin, Polynesian or Micronesian. Family members will feel the need to show up at the patient's bedside to demonstrate their concern, and even to stay with patients as long as possible to provide care and encouragement for the sick relative.

Referral to Other Specialists

Implications of Referral

There is an increased tendency for medicine to differentiate into various specialties associated with the expansion of medical knowledge and skill, and it is common practice that physicians will consult with and refer to other specialties. This was not true for traditional practice in the past, because the healer was supposed to be competent enough to know everything and to take care of every patient.

Therefore, to refer a patient to other specialties may be seen by the patient with traditional beliefs as evidence that the attending physician is not competent enough to understand and treat his or her medical problems, and thus needs another physician's help. Proper explanations may be needed for such situations. Many patients will understand and welcome being seen by other physicians who have special knowledge and experience.

Obtaining Psychiatric Consultation

Medical or surgical doctors may often encounter patients that they want to refer for a psychiatric consultation. In such cases, the physician may fear how the patient and his family perceive the meaning of having a *psychiatric* problem and how they understand the function of a psychiatrist. Most of the time, it is not the patient but the doctor who is uncomfortable about such a referral.

Doctors may fear that the patient will become angry with them, and ask if the doctor thinks they are *crazy*. The patient may also become anxious, fearful of a psychiatric evaluation. Actually, a little anxiety is not necessarily bad. The patient then pays more attention to his or her specific feelings, behaviors, and situation—sometimes even solving the particular issues at hand.

Generally speaking, psychiatric referral should be presented matter-of-factly. It is best to simply state that a psychiatric consultant is being called in to help the primary physician in his care for the patient. As long as the patient senses that the primary doctor is not abandoning him or her, the consultation is almost always accepted. Patients who reject a psychiatric consultation are often drug abusers, who fear that their ability to manipulate doctors into prescribing certain abusable medications will be diminished, and severely paranoid patients who suspect their caregivers are dishonest and malicious.

The culturally different may be unfamiliar with psychiatric care and have less of a stigma regarding it. They usually respect a physician's position of authority. The calling in of a consultant may be taken as an indication that the medical condition is being seen as important and is being seriously attended to. This, of course, depends upon the physician behaving confidently that calling in a psychiatric consultant is the right thing to do.

Discharge from the Hospital

Implication of Discharge

Discharge from a hospital is generally welcome because it is associated with the idea that the patient is now well enough to return home. However, some patients may feel insecure, thinking that they are not capable of caring for themselves or they fear their care will be inadequate at home. This is true for some patients who are discharged not because they have recovered from their illness but because there is no further treatment available. Sometimes it is due to the fact that the medical insurance may not cover their expenses anymore, and the patient cannot afford to stay longer. If the expense for hospitalization is taken care of by a public system (such as a national health care plan for certain groups, such as veterans), then there may be a struggle between the healthcare provider and the patient (and/or family) regarding the length of stay. Some patients may want to stay longer than is needed medically, or they may disagree that their medical needs for inpatient care have been met. These issues can shape the pattern of medical care as well.

Social factors will also determine the reaction to discharge from the hospital. If the patient is homeless, discharge means losing a warm bed, hot showers, and three meals a day. Such a patient may be very reluctant to leave the hospital. For some patients, discharge from the hospital implies loss of the sick role, with the expectation of resuming responsibilities in life or work. If they are not psychologically ready, they will be less than enthusiastic to leave the hospital. If the family is not willing or ready to take back the patient, the family will ask for a longer stay as well. Thus, discharge is not merely a medical issue—it has psychosocial and cultural overtones, also.

The influence of culture on inpatient discharge practices can be seen in the contrasting methods of treating myocardial infarction patients in Japan and in the United States. Hospital lengths of stay are three times longer in Japan, although days in the coronary care unit are similar (three days). In the United States, a significant period of post-hospital rehabilitation is usual. In Japan, however, most of the rehabilitation takes place in the hospital and the patient is much closer to returning to normal function at the time of discharge. In Japan, the determination of discharge is more flexible, and family members contribute a great deal to deciding that date (Muramatsu & Liang 1999). These differences are consistent with Eastern values of benevolent dependence among family or group members, versus Western values on individuality and autonomy (Doi 1973).

Follow-up

Every healthcare provider knows that follow-up care is important after discharge from the hospital. If the patient has a family doctor, continuous care is likely, so potentially fewer difficulties will arise. If care needs to be arranged after discharge, however, discharge planning becomes an important issue. The role of case managers or social workers can be critical in such cases to assure proper follow-up care.

In summary, the care of patients is not merely a matter of treating disease. Medical care is subject to various factors, including the patient's pre-existing medical condition, the patient's psychology, the family's attitude, available medical facilities, the social setting, the payment system, and cultural factors involving the patient, the physician, and the medical culture. To be culturally competent, health-care providers need to consider all these factors and be prepared to provide care that fits the social and cultural background of the patient in conjunction with the medical illness.

References

Ahmed I (2001) Psychological aspects of giving and receiving medications. In: Tseng WS, Streltzer J (eds) Culture and psychotherapy: A guide to clinical practice. Washington D.C. American Psychiatric Press, pp 123–134

Beyene Y (1992) Medical disclosure and refugees: Telling bad news to Ethiopian patients. Western Journal of Medicine 157:328–332

Buckalew LW, Coffield KE (1982) Drug expectations associated with perceptual characteristics: Ethnic factors. Perceptual and Motor Skills 55:915–918

Doi T (1973) The anatomy of dependence. Kodansha International, Tokyo

Giger JN, Davidhizar RE (eds) (1999) Transcultural Nursing: Assessment and Intervention, 3rd edn. Mosby, St. Louis

Gostin LO (1995) Informed consent, cultural sensitivity, and respect for persons. Journal of American Medical Association 274:844–845

Kandakai TL, Price JH, Telljiohann SK, Holiday-Goodman M (1996) Knowledge, beliefs, and use of prescribed antibiotic medications among low-socioeconomic African Americans. Journal of National Medical Association 88:289–294

Krauses-Mars AH, and Lachman P (1994) Breaking bad news to parents with disabled children: A cross-cultural study. Child Care, Health, and Development 20(2):101–113

Muramatsu N, Liang J (1999) Hospital length of stay in the United States and Japan: a case study of myocardial infarction patients. International Journal of Health Service 29:189–209

Novack DH, Plumer R, Smith RL, Ochitill H, Morrow GR, Bennett JM (1979) Changes in physicians' attitudes toward telling the cancer patient. Journal of American Medical Association 241:897–900

Nunley M (1996) Why psychiatrists in India prescribe so many drugs. Culture, Medicine and Psychiatry 20:165–97

Oken D (1961) What to tell cancer patients: a study of medical attitudes. Journal of American Medical Association 175:1120–1128

Racy J (1969) Death in an Arab couture. Annales of the New York Academy of Science 164:871–880

Tang LL, Bultz B, Zhang ZW, de Groot J (2006) The psychological reactions manifested by Chinese patients suffering from tumor: Cultural impact. The Proceeding of the First World Congress of Cultural Psychiatry S-II-20

Tavoli A, Mohagheghi MA, Montazeri A, Roshan R, Tavoli Z, Omidvari S (2007) Anxiety and depression in patients with gastrointestinal cancer: Does knowledge of cancer diagnosis matter? BMC Gastroenterology 7:28

Tse CY, Cong A, Fok SY (2003) Breaking bad news: A Chinese perspective. Palliative Medicine 17:339–343

Chapter 8
Culture and Special Medical Issues

In healthcare, there are various factors that impact the process of medical practice (as elaborated in the previous chapter). Besides medical knowledge, the medical setting, and socio-economic factors, there are cultural factors. In this chapter, we discuss cultural factors that influence various special medical issues that healthcare providers will encounter in the care of their patients.

Some Medically-Related Special Issues

Circumcision

Circumcision of boys is practiced worldwide. For Jews, it is an important religious custom to circumcise a male child soon after delivery, usually at home. Traditionally, a rabbi leads the prayers and performs the circumcision, although nowadays, a physician may be asked to perform the circumcision in the presence of the rabbi.

In some tribal cultures, circumcision is performed when a boy reaches puberty, to signify the entrance into adulthood. It is a painful experience, and the boy is taught to endure the process.

For years, it has been debated whether male circumcision has health benefits, particularly for a female partner. In some cultures, male circumcision is rare or infrequent, and evidence of health risks was not convincing. In the United States, the percent of males being circumcised has traditionally been high, but it has gradually declined. Recently, however, methodologically sound, large-scale studies in Africa have shown that the transmission of HIV/AIDS can be dramatically reduced by circumcision (Bailey 2007). Because of this new evidence of important health benefits from circumcision, health authorities will increasingly promote it worldwide. There is good evidence that cultural tradition can be overcome if the population is convinced of the safety of the procedure and the cost is minimal (Lukobo 2007).

W.-S. Tseng and J.M. Streltzer (eds.), *Cultural Competence in Health Care*
© Springer 2008

Genital Mutilation (Girls' Circumcision)

Female genital mutilation (FGM) is a traditional culture practice observed in some societies—particularly in Africa—even now. It is based on the cultural belief that females need to restrain their sexual desire and avoid sexual stimulation. The clitoris is amputated when the girl is young. It is a very painful procedure, seen by most people outside of these societies as a form of abuse against girls—one which affects their (sexual) lives as adult women later.

The practice is surprisingly common, with estimates of the prevalence of FGM as high as 137 million worldwide. Two million girls per year are considered at risk (Morrone, Hercogova & Lotti 2002). As international migration increases, so does the presence of circumcised women in Europe and other developed countries. Health education programs targeted at immigrant communities should include information on sexuality, FGM, and reproduction. Moreover, healthcare workers should discourage women from performing FGM on their daughters and help them to learn the codes of conduct and existing laws about the abuse of children.

Anuforo, Oyedele & Pacquiao (2004) examined beliefs about the practice of female circumcision among three main Nigerian ethnic tribes (Igbo, Yoruba, and Hausa) in the United States and Nigeria. They found that religion, education, and occupation were significant factors influencing attitudes toward continuation of the practice. They reported that government-sponsored public education and influence by media increased awareness of the complications of female circumcision.

Childhood Obesity

Obesity in children is increasing around the world, particularly in developed and developing societies. Excessive body weight can be attributed to multiple factors, including genetic predisposition, food intake patterns, physical exercise, and individual and cultural attitudes toward body size.

People in Asia, including children, tend to have slim physiques. However, there has been an increase in child obesity in Asian societies, including mainland China, Hong Kong, Japan, Korea, Singapore, and Taiwan. Associated with economic improvement and socio-cultural changes after World War II, the number of overweight children has increased so remarkably that clinics specifically designed for overweight children have been set up—a new phenomenon that was unheard of in those societies in the past. Several factors contribute to the new phenomenon of child obesity problems in these societies. There have been remarkable changes in food intake as the result of economic improvements. More nutritious food has become available and more meat is consumed than before. This has resulted in a higher calorie intake. This is in contrast to the lives of children before and during the war, when they often suffered from malnutrition due to a shortage of food.

In addition, physical exercise among children has decreased markedly. Associated with improvements in transportation, children seldom walk to school, as they did in the past even if many miles were required. Children used to participate in sports and outdoor games after school, or join their parents in doing household chores. Now, children increasingly watch TV, engage in electronic games, or study for school assignments because of heavy educational pressure. Lifestyles have changed greatly from several decades ago, and parents are facing new problems associated with these changes.

Child Abuse and Neglect

Child physical abuse and neglect are worldwide problems (Korbin 1981; Krugman 1996). Most studies that include ethnicity as a variable find it to be significant, although socio-economic factors seem to be primary (Miller & Cross 2006). Certain factors in the cultural context have been proposed to either increase the incidence of child abuse and neglect or to diminish the likelihood of their occurrence. These factors include the cultural value of children (whether children are viewed as valuable for future generations), beliefs about child capabilities and the developmental stages of children (expecting children to behave in certain ways at certain ages in terms of competence and humanness), how child-rearing is embedded in kin and community networks (the existence of a network of concerned individuals beyond the biological parents is a crucial element in the etiology of child abuse, and is also called *familism*) (Korbin 1981; Coohey 2001). While children might be highly valued in general by a cultural group, there are categories of children that are more vulnerable to maltreatment. These include illegitimate, adopted, deformed, retarded, high birth order, and female children. Vulnerability depends, to a large degree, on the cultural context.

From a clinical point of view, Maitra (1996) raised the question about a universal diagnostic category for child abuse. Based on cultural beliefs about the self, subjective experience, interpersonal connections, and child-rearing patterns, child abuse is viewed and defined differently in different societies. Special caution and careful assessment are thus necessary in transcultural practice.

Sexual Abuse

Even though it is suspected that sexual abuse of children by adults is not rare, the actual occurrence of this abuse is often concealed. It is not easy to obtain epidemiological data from communities regarding the prevalence of sexual abuse for cross-cultural comparison. A recent study of college students in Texas found that male and female students of Asian ancestry reported higher levels of physical and emotional abuse and neglect than their European counterparts. However, female students of European ancestry reported a higher incidence of sexual abuse than female students of Asian ancestry (Meston, Heiman, Trapnell & Carlin 1999). These results must be viewed cautiously, because the data was retrospective—examining childhood histories of the sexual abuse of adult subjects. Furthermore, college students are unlikely to be a representative population.

A study from the United Kingdom revealed that both professionals as well as lay people tended to deny the existence of sexual abuse of children among Asian ethnic minority populations, based on assumptions about the Asian family structure, its culture and its religion. It was noted that Asian family members were less likely to initiate concerns, and that professionals need to be more open to the possibility of sexual abuse (Moghal, Nota & Hobbs 1995). Immigrant youth—particularly those who experienced family disruption from traumatic circumstances—may be particularly at risk for sexual abuse. A study of young Hmong girls revealed very high rates of gang rape, prostitution, and multiple assaults (Edinburgh, Saewyc, Thao & Levitt 2006).

On the other hand, misunderstandings can lead to the accusation of sexual abuse where there is none, as in the following case example.

Case Example

A couple with a 5-year old daughter emigrated from Asia to the United States. Their English was very limited, but the wife was able to find a simple labor job outside of the house, leaving the husband to take care of the home. Their daughter developed a skin rash around her genital area, and was given some ointment by her pediatrician for local application. The father, who thought that it was his job to help the daughter apply the ointment, kindly did so, without thinking that it might be perceived as wrong to do so in the host society. At the daughter's kindergarten, as part of a routine exercise, the teacher gave a picture to all the students, inquiring if any person had touched their *private* places. The teacher was surprised to learn from this particular girl that her father touched her private place *every day*. The alarmed teacher reported this to child protection services, and the social worker, accompanied by a policeman, went to the house intending to remove the girl for her *protection*. Without knowing what was going on, the father panicked and tried to stop his daughter from being taken away. He physically struggled with the police. In the middle of the physical conflict, the policeman drew his gun—perhaps trying to stop the father's desperate, violent behavior—and by mistake, shot the father. The mother came back from work and was shocked to discover her daughter in a state of panic and her husband dead (Tseng 2003, pp 282–283). The tragedy of this case might have been avoided if the social worker had consulted the pediatrician regarding any history or risk of sexual abuse of the child, rather than deciding to immediately take action using the police. A proper interpreter may have helped communicate adequate explanations between the family and the professional to avoid this unfortunate result.

Pain Management

Pain is one of the most common complaints made by patients. However, pain is a difficult somatic complaint to assess due to its entirely subjective nature. The complaint of pain is subject to the patient's personality, innate tolerance of pain, attitude toward pain, style of presenting suffering to others, and possible gains for presenting such suffering. There is wide individual variation in the response to pain stimuli. The cultural background of the patient can be influential in this regard (Streltzer 1997).

Pain researchers have shown interest in whether pain varies by ethnic group. Perhaps the most well-known study relating culture to pain was published by Zborowski (1952). He concluded that responses to painful illness were related to the patient's ethnic group. He described *old Americans* (Anglo-Saxon Protestants who had lived in the United States for several generations) as being stoic in response to their pain. Italians and Jews, in contrast, did not hesitate to complain openly about their pain. The Italians wanted immediate pain relief, whereas the Jews were fearful of medication that would take away their pain. The interpretation was that they wanted to be able to monitor their pain, which they perceived as a sign of how their illness was doing. This paper presented conclusions only, without any data. It may have been consistent with prevalent stereotypes.

Zborowski's study was followed by more sophisticated studies, whose results were not as dramatic, but did reveal subtle differences. For instance, Woodrow, Freidman, Siegelaub and Collen (1972) studied experimental pain in over 40,000 patients who were obtaining routine health screening in California. Pressure was applied to the Achilles tendon with a vise-like apparatus. They reported that Caucasian-Americans tolerated more pain than African-Americans, who in turn tolerated more pain than Asian-Americans.

To study acute clinical pain, Streltzer and Wade (1981) examined surgery patients undergoing elective gall bladder removal in the multi-ethnic society of Hawaii. Caucasian-Americans received the most post-operative pain medication. Filipino-Americans, Japanese-Americans, and Chinese-Americans received least, while Hawaiian-Americans were intermediate. In trying to explain this result, the ethnicities of the surgeons were identified. It was discovered that surgeon's orders were almost identical (according to the medical custom of the time) irrespective of ethnic group. The difference in treatment appeared to be at the level of nurse-patient interaction. The patients of Asian background were less vocal in complaining of pain to the nurses. In the medical culture at the time the study was done, undertreatment of acute pain was the norm, and the nurses may have felt that giving fewer narcotics meant better nursing care. Perhaps the patients of Asian background were more eager to please their nurses.

Stereotyping is a danger when healthcare personnel evaluate a patient's pain. It is easy to give more attention to someone from a more verbal and expressive culture, and to conclude that pain is more severe, or less well-tolerated. In fact, however, there is more variation due to individual factors in pain perception than that caused by cultural background. Furthermore, the trends of medical practice in the community will most strongly determine the actual pain treatment.

The prevailing medical culture greatly influences the treatment of painful conditions. For example, the degree of lower back pain and the related psychosocial dysfunction may not correlate at all with physical findings explaining the pain, and this fact varies substantially by country (Sanders, Brena, Spier, Beltrutti, McConnell & Quintero 1992). Some of this may be directly related to the culture of the society, and some of it may be related to the medical care system, including the presence of entitlements for disability.

The following case example is not uncommon in the United States, and can occur in other countries, such as Denmark, Australia, and the United Kingdom. It would be practically unheard of, however, in China, Japan, or Italy.

Case Example

A 48-year old woman had been the manager of a convenience store for several years. She worked long hours for relatively low pay. She developed lower back pain one day after routinely lifting some boxes. She went to a physician who authorized disability leave from work for two weeks, and prescribed an opioid pain medication. After two weeks, she complained that the pain was no better. Leave was extended, and the dose of medication increased. Over time, she had many unrevealing diagnostic tests, and she failed to improve despite numerous types of treatments. She became dependent on high doses of opioids, which did not improve her condition, but which she insisted she could not do without. She eventually received permanent disability benefits.

Issues Relating to Surgery

Most people appreciate that surgery can be effective in treating certain medical conditions, such as appendicitis, and may even be needed to save one's life. However, based on unique cultural beliefs, some patients may have specific psychological reactions to certain surgical procedures, such as those that result in the loss of a part of the body. To lose a part of one's body may be interpreted as a loss of one's integrity. Influenced by such a belief, a diabetic patient may refuse amputation of a leg that is necrotic from ulcers, or a woman with breast cancer may choose chemotherapy rather than surgical removal of her breast, even though it may result in a lower rate of cure.

Case Example

An Asian diabetic patient refused to amputate his leg, despite a life-threatening condition. In this case, a culturally appropriate solution was found by the medical staff. The amputated limb would be stored in a freezer to be able to retrieve it for burial with the body at the time of death in the future

Cesarian Section

In obstetrics, birth by cesarean section has become increasingly widespread in many countries. In Australia, the percentageof births by cesarean section has risen from 17 percent in 1990 to 23 percent in 2000. A survey of post-partum women indicated that 71.4 percent agreed that cesarean section offers an easier way of giving birth, and an elective cesarean section was considered by almost 15 percent of women (Walker, Turnbull & Wilkinson 2004), showing that the community attitude toward this surgical operation was changing, with the perception of cesarean section as an easy and convenient way of giving birth.

Blood Transfusion

When a person loses a lot of blood, either from external trauma or internal bleeding, blood transfusion becomes necessary. Blood transfusions are also sometimes necessary during surgery. While it is common for people to be concerned about how much blood will be lost during an operation, in some cultures, blood is considered particularly vital and there might be a strong wish to conserve it as much as possible. In such a case, there might be less opposition toward receiving blood transfusions to gain the needed vital body fluid. In contrast, certain religions—such as Jehovah's Witnesses—might lead thier members to refuse to accept a blood transfusion, even as a life-saving treatment.

The followers of Jehovah's Witnesses, based on their interpretation of the (Christian) bible, understand that blood is not to be consumed. Therefore, they consider that it is wrong to have blood transfused. They accept the transfusion of plasma, but not fluid that contains blood cells. They promote alternative ways to deal with the medical consequences of blood loss.

It is a serious medical dilemma when a blood transfusion is required to save patient's life, yet the patient (or the patient's guardian) is a member of Jehovah's Witnesses and refuses to authorize the procedure. Legal remedies have been sought, and there have been several instances where a judge has ordered the administration of the needed blood transfusion (Tseng, Mathews & Elwyn 2004, pp 278–279).

Case Example

A 58-year old man was diagnosed with colon cancer. His surgeon wanted to operate, and the patient agreed to surgery as long as no blood transfusion would be done because it was against the principles of his religion as a Jehovah's Witness. The surgeon was disturbed by this request, not wanting to be limited in any way in his surgical decisions. He decided he would not perform surgery unless a psychiatric consultant could impress upon the patient the possibility that a transfusion may be necessary during the operation, and get him to change his mind. The consultant discovered that the patient had been hospitalized for schizophrenia several times prior to the age of 30. He then converted to Jehovah's Witnesses, and for the first time in his life had a very supportive family-like social network. He was able to obtain a job as a janitor, and eventually get married. He believed that he owed everything of value in his life to his religion, and he would not compromise on the issue of a blood transfusion. The psychiatric consultant then wondered what the risks versus the benefits would be if surgery were performed without the possibility of a transfusion. If surgery was potentially life-saving, with relatively little life-threatening risk, perhaps the surgical team could be convinced to go ahead and operate despite the less-than-ideal circumstances. As it turned out, the surgical team could not state what the chances were for a cure, and what the likelihood of a life-threatening bleed during surgery might be. The team agreed to investigate this further, and ultimately determined that chances for a cure were not good, and little better than chemotherapy alone. Surgery was not worth doing under the best of circumstances.

Organ Donation and Transplantation

In spite of the remarkable medical technology that now exists for organ transplantations, relatively few people volunteer to donate their organs after death. The low rate of organ donation is supported among some ethnic groups, such as Hispanics (Frates & Garcia Bohrere 2002), Asian-Americans (Albright, Glanz, Wong, Dela Cruz, Abe & Sagayadoro 2005). Lack of medical knowledge, a reluctance to discuss death, and the belief that a body should be preserved intact are some of the major cultural factors limiting organ donation (Molzahn, Starzomski, McDonald & O'Loughlin 2005).

The severe donor shortage, which limits transplantation as a lifesaving treatment, causes an ethical dilemma. Criteria for distribution of organs for patients waiting for transplantation are the subject of continuing debate. By law, age, race, and socio-economic status cannot play a role, yet determining the risks and benefits for medically ill patients can be a complex medical assessment and an ethical conundrum (Markmann, Brayman, Naji, Ohthoff, Shaked & Barker 2004, p 750). Needless to say, the decision will be subject to the impact of social and cultural values, including the medical culture of the times.

Due to the shortage of organs for transplantation, healthy poor people in developing societies are selling their organs (usually kidneys). The sale of organs in a commercial manner has serious ethical ramifications. This practice is condemned by the International Transplantation Society and is forbidden by law in most Western countries (Markmann, Brayman, Naji, Olthoff, Shaked & Barker 2004).

In the United States, donor authorizations tend to be especially low among African-Americans and other minority ethnic groups. Rubens (1996) carried out a questionnaire survey of the beliefs and attitudes toward organ transplantation and rates of participation regarding organ donation among a sample of racially and eth-nically mixed university students at a state university in the midwestern United States. He reported that African-American students differed significantly from Caucasian students in their attitudes and beliefs toward organ donation. However, a greater percentage of African-American students granted permission for organ donation than African-Americans in the general population.

Among the various reasons that people are reluctant about organ donation is the cultural view that it is very important to keep the whole body intact, even for burial or cremation. Regarding Chinese-Canadians, Molzahn, Starzomski, McDonald, and O'Loughlin (2005) reported that, in addition to the basic belief that it is impor-tant to preserve an intact body, lack of medical knowledge and communication about organ donation and concerns about the possible influence of spiritual or cul-tural values are other factors contributing to the obstacle for organ donation. In the Islamic religion, a Muslim does not own his or her body but holds it in a *trust from God*. Consequently, a Muslim cannot donate or receive organs, and blood transfu-sions are permissible only if recommended by a physician who is Muslim for the purpose of saving that person from death. Similarly, American Indians traditionally view a dead body as a seed that is placed in the ground. Just as a seed is planted whole, so the body should be buried intact.

From a patient's perspective, receiving an organ transplant may have a major psychological impact. For example, in Asia a criminal agreed to donate his organs and cornea before he was executed. This *good deed* was publicized. However, in spite of this, many patients who were on the waiting list for some time for liver, kidney, and cornea transplants refused to receive the organs because they were coming from a criminal.

Chinese patients in Taiwan who need organ transplantation strongly prefer to receive an organ donated from immediate family rather than from a *stranger*. It becomes a family member's duty to donate the organ to their relative who needs a transplant. Often aged parents will donate an organ to an adult child. The family will strongly oppose physician's suggestion to use an organ from an unrelated other person (Yeh 2000).

In Italy, remarkable cultural changes have occurred relative to pediatric cardiac transplantation in the last twenty years. The changes have been associated with a different approach to the donation of organs, technical progress, collaboration of interdisciplinary teams, and greater attention to the psychological aspects of the patient. Attitudes toward cardiac transplantation have become much more accept-ing, and the total number of cases receiving cardiac transplants has increased with good survival rate (Bioni, Rossi, De Ranieri, Tabarini, Mira & Parisi 2006).

Sterilization, Hysterectomy, and Artificial Insemination

Continuing the family line is an important concern for people of many cultures, with blood-related descendents the desired way to maintain the family line. To adopt a child from a nonblood-related person is the less preferred way. Based on this cultural concept, medical procedures related to the matter of reproduction may have a strong psychological impact on the patient, spouse, and family, if they hold strong beliefs about the continuity of the family line.

Sterilization

From a medical point of view, sterilization is a simple surgical operation and a way of family planning. Yet, there may be a significant psychological impact depending on how such a procedure is viewed by the patient's culture. In some cultures, particularly those that strongly emphasize the need for many children, sterilization can be seen as a very unwelcome procedure. From a technical perspective, male sterilization is much easier, with fewer complications than female sterilization by tubal ligation or hysterectomy (Cunningham Leveno, Bloom, Hauth, Gilstrap & Wenstrom 2005, pp 755–776). However, for a society that emphasizes a superior role for men, sterilization of men may be considered almost equal to castration, even though medically it is not. Sterilization of women is more favorably accepted by their male partners in such cultures.

Hysterectomy

In many cultures, reproduction is considered one of the major functions of women, and losing the uterus is equivalent to losing the power of being a woman. Many women fear a change in sexual desire after a hysterectomy, and that their husbands will not want them because they are *incomplete* as a woman. There is a great concern that the husband may want to abandon or divorce her, or insist upon having another wife or a concubine to bear his children. As a result, a woman might refuse to have her uterus removed, and she might develop anxiety and depression after a hysterectomy.

Artificial Insemination

Artificial insemination is a medical procedure that can be used to help certain women bear children. If the husband's semen is used, there are fewer psychological complications. However, if semen from another donor is used, this may become a great issue—especially in a society in which it is very important to have child of one's own blood. The psychological acceptance of such procedure by the husband, or by the immediate family, may be a significant issue.

Abortion and Infanticide

In addition to bearing children, the artificial ending of a child's (or potential child's) life is also subject to different reactions from various cultures. Some cultures tolerate it, or even accept it as a part of life, and others oppose such action as equivalent to baby-killing.

Abortion

To terminate the life of a fetus via an induced or artificial abortion is the subject of intense emotional, political, and ethical debate in many countries. In the United States, there is no foreseeable resolution to the conflict, which has involved radical acts such as the bombing of abortion clinics and the shooting of physicians who perform abortions. However, in many countries, abortion is an accepted part of family planning. This is particularly true in societies that accept the concept of population control. To give birth to a baby without being married is considered shameful in many cultures. In such cases, abortion will be a common choice for a woman who becomes pregnant outside of marriage. Thus, abortion is not merely a medical choice, but also a social, cultural, and political matter.

In the United States, the rate of induced abortion per 1,000 population is highest for African-American women (57.4), intermediate for Hispanic women (30.6), and lowest for non-Hispanic Caucasian women (11.7) (Hamilton & Ventura 2006), demonstrating considerably different rates among different ethnic groups. Artificial abortion has been actively used as a means for family control in states of the former Soviet Union. In Kazakhstan, despite an overall decline in abortion and increase in contraceptive use since independence in 1991, abortion has remained a prominent part of the country's reproductive culture and practices (Agadjanian 2002).

The extent that it is psychologically traumatic for women to go through induced abortion is associated with the society's attitude toward such. In a study comparing American women with Russian women, 14.3 percent of American women, and only 0.9 percent of Russian women experienced post-traumatic stress disorders after an induced abortion (Rue, Coleman, Rue & Reardon 2004). Russian women had a much more liberal attitude toward this procedure.

Latina women have often been portrayed as holding strong traditional family values, leading to a greater propensity for rejection of contraception and abortion. A study of 1,207 ever-pregnant young Latina women aged 14–24 recruited at family planning clinics in Los Angeles found that only a small portion (7.5%) of the young women had ever had an induced abortion. The variables significantly associated with past abortion included less traditional attitudes about women's roles, higher gravidity, and a higher number of lifetime sexual partners. The conclusion was that use of abortion among Latinas is driven by role orientation and reproductive variables (Kaplan, Erickson, Stewart & Crane 2001).

To explore traditional Hmong explanations about abortion and practices that pertain to it, Liamputtong (2003) conducted interviews with Hmong living in Melbourne, Australia. It was found that Hmong women are knowledgeable about fertility control methods, including abortion, but only women who are older and have had many children to ensure the continuity of the lineage are considered to have the right to abortion—younger women do not have this right. The culture values having many children, and abortion is not easily accepted because it upsets the cosmological balance of the society. This has clinical implications because it affects younger Hmong women who may wish to control their fertility.

An ethnographic study of midwives in the rural township of Morelos, Mexico found that midwives viewed miscarriage as a woman's failure to fulfill her primary role as mother, and they viewed induced abortion as a grave sin or crime (Castaneda, Billings & Blanco 2003). Nevertheless, under certain circumstances, many midwives could justify the practice of induced abortion. Helping women to *let down the period* in situations when a woman's menstrual period was delayed was acceptable to midwives, as it was not viewed as abortion but enabling women to regain health and well-being.

In Thailand (a Buddhist society), abortion is illegal, except in cases when it is considered necessary for a women's health, or in the case of rape. However, in reality, abortion is common in Thailand (Whittaker 2002). Within the restrictive legal context, risk is stratified along economic lines. Poorer women have little choice but to resort to abortion to reduce their family size. Untrained practitioners are used for the abortion because licensed physicians dare not carry out such due to the risk of legal punishment.

Infanticide

To end the life of a baby after birth sounds like a cruel and criminal act. Yet, infanticide has been carried out in many cultures in the past, and even now in some societies. For instance, in Japan, the custom of killing unwanted babies was a common practice in the past (particularly for poor farmers). The folk name for this practice was *mabuki*, (implying a need to remove extra plants to make space for other plants). In those days, without family planning, excess children were a financial burden to poor farmers, who carried out such practice. In many cultures, a handicapped baby is killed because it would have difficulty surviving, and it is rationalized that it is best to *return* the infant to nature. Conflict thus occurs among medical, cultural, and legal issues (Tseng, Matthews & Elwyn 2004, pp 147–153).

Adjustment to Aging

Adjustment to the changes inherent in growing old is the major task of the elderly. Loss, in particular, is an inevitable part of aging, and includes loss of physical capabilities, occupational status, and, most importantly, the loss of spouse, family, or friends. A positive adjustment to aging is found in those who can feel that their life has been worthwhile and in those who willingly and consciously adapt to change. The ease of adjustment to aging can be very much influenced by the prevailing social and cultural attitudes toward aging, as well as attitudes toward death. Societies vary in their respect for the elderly, provision of care, and attitude toward the importance of helping the elderly age comfortably. The elderly use family physicians for more than just medical care. They are more willing to discuss their innermost feelings about aging-related issues with their doctors (Brummel-Smith & Mosqueda 2003, p 14).

Death and Dying

Even though death, from a narrow perspective, is primarily a biological phenomenon—i.e., the end of the life of an organism—it is associated greatly with psychological matters. Death can have many meanings: it can be seen merely as a biological event, a rite of passage, an inevitable natural occurrence, or many other things. Needless to day, culture contributes to the perspectives on death and dying (Ross 1981).

In many African traditions, elders take on an important new status through death, joining the ancestors who watch over their own descendants, as well as those of the entire village. Therefore, everyone in the village participates in a funeral to prepare the deceased's journey to the ancestral realm. The death of the individual becomes an occasion for the affirmation of the entire community, as members jointly celebrate their connection with each other and with their collective past.

In contrast, in many Muslim societies, death affirms faith in God (Allah). People are taught that the achievements, problems, and pleasures of this life are transitory and ephemeral, and that everyone should be mindful of, and ready for, death at any time. In Buddhist societies such as Thailand, based on their religious thoughts of reincarnation, the present life is considered part of a whole—a circulating cycle. Death is simply an entrance to another part of the cycle. In Hindu societies, such as India, helping the dying to relinquish their ties to this world and prepare for the next is a particularly important obligation for the immediate family.

From the examples just mentioned above, it is clear that attitudes toward death, and reactions to the loss of a close person, are shaped by religious thought or philosophy of life. However, when we look at how the individual actually feels and deals with his predicament, the suffering individual is not content with theological thought or philosophical explanation. Even within any one religious denomination, there can be many different explanations of the meaning of death that are reflected in that group's characteristic ways of grieving. This is illustrated by the variety that exists within Christian groups (Eisenbruch 1984).

In the past, throughout most of Western society, death was an accepted, familiar event that usually occurred at home. In 20th century North America and Western Europe, death came to be withdrawn from everyday life. More and more people died alone in hospitals rather than at home among family members.

Helping a patient face death, and planning for important issues after death, is a part of the work of healthcare providers. It is thus important to know how to approach the subject of death with patients and their families. Perkins, Shepard, Cortez & Hazuda (2005) explored attitudes about discussing death and postmortem medical procedure among chronically ill seniors in San Antonio, Texas. They found that attitudes about discussing death differed between ethnic groups. Mexican-Americans and Caucasian-Americans favored such discussions, but African-Americans did not. Regarding postmortem procedures—such as organ donation, autopsy, and practice on cadavers—Mexican-Americans viewed the procedure most favorably, Caucasian-Americans less so, and African-Americans least so.

Ending Life

Although it is a universal desire for a person to live as long as possible and to find ways to prolong life, attitudes toward death are subject to cultural influences. Prolonging life through intensive care or by mechanical means may not be appreciated in all cultures. In some, it is considered a good and natural phenomenon to die after a certain age, and death may be treated as a happy occasion rather than a sad one. From a healthcare point of view, it is the caregiver's role to help the patient have a *good* death, with more comfort and less suffering.

In many cultures, it is considered desirable for people to die in their own homes surrounded by their immediate family members. When this is the custom, the family may ask the physician about the prognosis of the patient's medical condition to plan for this eventuality. If the patient is considered to have no hope for recovery, it becomes the physician's responsibility to inform the family of the appropriate time for the patient to be discharged from the hospital so that his last days may be spent at home.

Legal Definition of Death

The medical and legal definition of *death* is not uniform around the world. In the United States, *brain death*—as verified by an electroencephalogram (EEG)—is sufficient to determine death legally. In contrast, Japan is more conservative, defining *death* as the complete stopping of the heartbeat. These different ways of defining *legal* death have a direct impact on organ donation.

In 1997, a newspaper in Hawaii (*The Honolulu Advertiser*) reported a story about an 8-year old Japanese girl who received $600,000 in donations in Japan for a badly needed heart transplant, but had to come to the United States for the operation. The tight legal definition of death in Japan made it very difficult to obtain a suitable heart for transplantation. Two years later, after many years of struggle between the professional and legal systems, Japan finally passed a law that brain death would be accepted as the criterion for death to facilitate organ donation. Heart transplants then occurred successfully in Japan, but only rarely—17 between 1999 and 2003 (Osada & Imaizumi 2005).

Grief and Mourning

Although the loss of a significant person in life is always an emotional event, there is a diversity of customs sanctioned by different cultures for people to guide their reactions when they experience a close person's death. The survivors' grief reactions may start when a patient dies in the hospital. Healthcare providers can perform an important service for the survivors by recognizing and facilitating their culturally-sanctioned grief reactions. Therefore, it is useful for healthcare professionals to know how different cultures manage the period of grief.

According to the customs of orthodox Jews, relatives must remain with a dying family member so that the soul does not leave while the person is alone. Leaving a dead body unattended would be a sign of disrespect (Rabinowicz 1979). In the Jewish tradition, those who are making condolence visits are advised to enter the house and sit silently unless the mourners show a desire to speak of their loss.

Physician-Assisted Suicide and Euthanasia

Associated with advances in healthcare that extend life, there is an increased likelihood that a state of deteriorating physical or mental health can develop—especially for some elderly. In these cases, the possibility of actively ending someone's life has become a consideration. Physician-assisted suicide and euthanasia have become controversial topics in many societies (Coomaraswamy 1996). One can distinguish between *active* and *passive* euthanasia. In the former, the physician takes an active role, using medical means to end the life of a person wishing to die. In the latter, the physician withdraws all medical methods of sustaining a person's life so that the person will eventually die.

After reviewing situations in Germany, Holland, and the United States, Battin (1991) pointed out that, although they are alike in that their aging populations die primarily of deteriorative diseases, end-of-life dilemmas were handled differently in these three countries. In the United States (at that time), withholding and withdrawing of treatment were the only legally recognized means of aiding the process of dying. In Holland, voluntary active euthanasia has been practiced by physicians. In Germany, assisted suicide has been a legal option, but is usually practiced outside of a medical setting.

Clearly, the way we deal with a person wishing to end his life is a complicated issue that needs to be carefully thought about and decided upon. It involves philosophical, practical, medical, legal, and cultural matters for which answers are not always present. From a clinical point of view, a patient who expresses the desire for euthanasia may be manifesting a depressive illness, unhappiness because of interpersonal conflict, or even misunderstandings about his or her clinical course and prognosis. Therefore, it is a good idea to have psychiatric consultation to assess the mental condition of patients with an expressed wish for euthanasia.

Autopsy

To clarify the reason for death (either medically or for forensic purposes), and to increase medical knowledge, an autopsy of a deceased person may be performed. If the autopsy is mandatory due to forensic reasons, the family has no right to refuse such procedure. However, if it is not, agreement from the family is necessary. This can cause an awkward situation if the family refuses to allow an autopsy on the patient, even if such is indicated medically.

In accordance with the common belief that the body should be kept intact after death, it may be difficult to obtain agreement from the surviving family for an autopsy of the deceased. In many cultures, it is almost impossible to obtain permission for an autopsy unless it is legally required. The autopsy rate in Arab countries is extremely low, and cadavers are not permitted for use in teaching or research purposes. This is also true in many Asian countries, where the family is not keen about the idea of autopsy, and cadavers for medical teaching often come only from homeless people who die without family. It is certainly a challenge for physicians to persuade the surviving family to permit an autopsy in such cultures.

This chapter has discussed the cultural aspects of various special issues relating to medical practice. It is intended to increase awareness of the broad range of issues that can be influenced by culture. The ones mentioned in this chapter are far from exhaustive. The examples given are not part of a specific list of cultural situations. Rather, every patient should be viewed as having a cultural background that may be important in the medical care provided in many medical situations.

References

Agadjanian V (2002) Is "abortion culture" fading in the former Soviet Union? Views about abortion and contraception in Kazakhstan. Studies in Family Planning 33:237–48

Albright CL, Glanz K, Wong L, Dela Cruz MR, Abe L, Sagayadora TL (2005) Knowledge and attitudes about decreased donor organ donation in Filipinos: A qualitative assessment. Transplantation Proceedings 37: 4153–4158

Anuforo PO, Oyedele L, Pacquiao DF (2004) Comparative study of meanings, beliefs, and practices of female circumcision among three Nigerian tribes in the United States and Nigeria. Journal of Transcultural Nursing 15:103–113

Bailey RC, Moses S, Parker CB, Agot K, Maclean I, Krieger JN, Williams CF, Campbell RT, Ndinya-Achola JO (2007) Male circumcision for HIV prevention in young men in Kisumu, Kenya: A randomised controlled trial. Lancet 369(9562):643–56

Battin MP (1991) Euthanasia: The way we do it, the way they do it. Journal of Pain Symptom Management 6(5):298–305

Biondi G, Rossi A, De Ranieri C, Tabarini P, Mira M, Parisi F (2006) Cultural Changes in Pediatric Heart Transplants: Twenty Years' Experience. The Proceeding of the First World Congress of Cultural Psychiatry, S-II-20

Brummel-Smith K, Mosqueda L (2003) Stages of human development. In: Taylor RB (ed) Family Medicine: Principles and Practice Springer, New York, pp 10–16

Castaneda X, Billings DL, Blanco J (2003) Abortion beliefs and practices among midwives (parteras) in a rural Mexican township. Womens Health 37(2):73–87

Coohey C (2001) The relationship between familism and child maltreatment in Latino and Anglo families. Child Maltreatment 6:130–42

Coomaraswamy RP (1994) Death, dying, and assisted suicide. Connecticut Medicine 58(9):551–556

Cunningham FG, Leveno KJ, Bloom SL, Hauth JC, Gilstrap L III, Wenstrom KD (2005) Willams Obstetrics, 22nd edn. McGraw-Hill, New York

Edinburgh L, Saewyc E, Thao T, Levitt C (2006) Sexual exploitation of very young Hmong girls. Journal of Adolescent Health 39:111–8

Eisenbruch M (1984) Cross-cultural aspects of bereavement. II: Ethnic and cultural variations in the development of bereavement practice. Culture, Medicine and Psychiatry 8(4):315–347

Frates J, Garcia Bohrere G (2002) Hispanic perception of organ donation. Progress in Transplantation 12(3):169–175

Hamilton BE, Ventura SJ (2006) Fertility and abortion rates in the United States, 1960–2002. International Journal of Andrology 29:34–45

Kaplan CP, Erickson PI, Stewart SL, Crane LA (2001) Young Latinas and abortion: the role of cultural factors, reproductive behavior, and alternative roles to motherhood. Healthcare for Women International 22(7):667–89

Korbin JE (ed) (1981) Child Abuse and Neglect: Cross-cultural Perspectives. University of California Press, Berkeley

Krugman RD (1996) Child abuse and neglect: A worldwide problem. In: Mak FL, Nadelson CC (eds) International Review of Psychiatry, vol 2. American Psychiatric Press, Washington D.C., pp 367–377

Liamputtong P (2003) Abortion—it is for some women only! Hmong women's perceptions of abortion. Healthcare for Women International 24:230–41

Lukobo MD, Bailey RC (2007) Acceptability of male circumcision for prevention of HIV infection in Zambia. AIDS Care 19:471–7

Maitra B (1996) Child abuse: A universal diagnostic category? The implication of culture in definition and assessment. International Journal of Social Psychiatry 42:287–304

Markmann JF, Brayman KL, Naji A, Olthoff KM, Shaked A, Barker CF (2004) Transplantation of abdominal organs, p. 750 In: Townsend CM, Beauchamp ED, Evers BM, and Mattox KL (eds) Sabiston textbook of surgery: The biological basis of modern surgical practice, 17th edn. Elsevier, Philadelphia, pp 699–755

Meston CM, Heiman JR, Trapnell PD, Carlin AS (1999) Ethnicity, desirable responding, and self-reports of abuse: A comparison of European- and Asian-ancestry undergraduates. Journal of Counseling and Clinical Psychology 67:139–144

Miller AB, Cross T (2006) Ethnicity in child maltreatment research: A replication of Behl et al.'s content analysis. Child Maltreatment 11:16–26

Moghal NE, Nota IK, Hobbs CJ (1995) A study of sexual abuse in an Asian community. Archives of Diseases in Childhood 72:346–347

Molzahn AE, Starzomski R, McDonald M, O'Loughlin C (2005) Chinese Canadian beliefs toward organ donation. Qualitative Health Research 15(1):82–98

Morrone A, Hercogova J, Lotti T (2002) Stop female genital mutilation: appeal to the international dermatologic community. International Journal of Dermatology 41:253–63

Osada K, Imaizumi T (2005) Special report from the Heart Transplant Candidate Registry Committee in Japan. The Journal of Heart and Lung Transplantation 24:810–814

Perkins HS, Shepherd KJ, Cortez JD, Hazuda HP (2005) Exploring chronically ill seniors' attitudes about discussing death and postmortem medical procedures. Journal of the American Geriatrics Society 53(5):895–900

Rabinowicz H (1979) Care of the terminal patient: The Jewish view of death. Nursing Times 75(18):757

Ross HM (1981) Societal/cultural views regarding death and dying. Topics in Clinical Nursing 3(3):1–16

Rubens AJ (1996) Racial and ethnic differences in students' attitudes and behavior toward organ donation. Journal of National Medical Association 88(7):417–421

Rue VM, Coleman PK, Rue J J, Reardon DC (2004) Induced abortion and traumatic stress: a preliminary comparison of American and Russian women. Medical Science of Monitoring 10(10):SR5–16

Sanders SH, Brena SF, Spier CJ, Beltrutti D, McConnell H, Quintero O (1992) Chronic low back pain patients around the world: cross-cultural similarities and differences. Clinical Journal of Pain 8:317–23

Streltzer J (1997) Pain. In: Tseng WS, Streltzer J (eds) Culture and psychopathology: A guide to clinical assessment. Brunner/Mazel, New York

Streltzer J, Wade TC (1981) The influence of cultural group on the undertreatment of postoperative pain. Psychosomatic Medicine 43:397–403

Tseng WS (2003) Clinician's Guide to Cultural Psychiatry. Academic Press, San Diego

Tseng WS, Matthews D, Elwyn TS (2004) Cultural Competence in Forensic Mental Health: A Guide for Psychiatrists, Psychologists, and Attorneys. Brunner-Routledge, New York

Walker R, Turnbull D, Wilkinson C (2004) Increasing cesarean section rates: Exploring the role of culture in an Australian community. Birth 31(2):117–124

Whittaker A (2002) Reproducing inequalities: Abortion policy and practice in Thailand. Womens Health 35(4):101–19

Wikipedia (2007). Jehovah's Witnesses and Blood. http://en.wikipedia.org/wiki/Jehovah's_ Witnesses#Blood accessed Dec. 1, 2007

Woodrow KM, Freidman GD, Siegelaub AB, Collen MF (1972) Pain tolerance: Differences according to age, sex and race. Psychosomatic Medicine 34:548–556

Yeh EK (2000) Personal communication.

Zborowski M (1952) Cultural components in responses to pain. Journal of Social Issues 8:16–30

Chapter 9
Conclusions

Relevance of Focusing on Culture

Cultural competence is an ideal to be strived for. The cultural aspects of medical practice and healthcare in general are legion, although the significance of cultural factors can vary greatly depending on the particular patient and the type of medical problem. In principle, the more purely biological the problem, the less there is a need to emphasize the cultural dimension—while the more that psychological and behavioral issues intersect with and are part of the medical problems, the greater the importance of cultural issues becomes.

For instance, in the case of acute traumatic injury, healthcare providers in the emergency department need to pay attention to the location of the injury and degree of damage, vital signs, laboratory tests and imaging, immediate management including intravenous access, possible blood transfusion, and so forth, and possible preparations for surgery. This is mainly a *medical* matter, with cultural factors playing little role. However, when it becomes necessary to explain to the patient that surgery is needed, or that a part of the body may be removed, or that physical rehabilitation may be needed, then healthcare provider-patient communication is involved and a relationship develops. Psychological and behavioral issues matter in medical situations, and these involve social and cultural issues. Consequently, even for the same patient with the same medical problem, the focus may change at a different stage of management.

It is also true that certain medical diseases or conditions need more focus on *medical* aspects, while others need more *psychological* and *sociocultural* attention. For instance, appendicitis, acute pancreatitis, and myocardial infarction may need medical attention predominantly (at least in the acute stage), while child abuse, obesity, venereal disease, and abortion may need more psychological attention with consideration of cultural issues.

W.-S. Tseng and J.M. Streltzer (eds.), *Cultural Competence in Health Care*
© Springer 2008

Characteristics of the Culturally Competent Provider

Cultural Sensitivity

Several basic qualities are required to become a culturally competent healthcare provider (Tseng 2003, pp 219–225). The clinician needs to have a basic cultural sensitivity. This means that the clinician can to be sensitive to, aware of, and have an appreciation for the existence of various lifestyles among human beings, with their diverse views and attitudes toward patterns of living, different types of stress endured, and varying coping patterns for adaptation. Actual experience encountering cultures other than one's own can facilitate and stimulate the development of cultural awareness and sensitivity.

Beyond a general awareness, the clinician needs to be perceptive enough to be able to sense cultural differences among people and know how to appreciate them without ignorance, bias, prejudice, or stereotyping. The clinician or care provider needs to be willing to communicate and learn as much as possible from his patients and their families about their beliefs, attitudes, value systems, and their ways of thinking and dealing with problems. It is not merely a matter of sensitive perception, but is also an attitude of wanting to learn about and understand others' lifestyles rather than being trapped in one's own subjective perception and interpretation of others' behavior.

Cultural Knowledge

Beyond sensitivity, a clinician needs to have a certain base of cultural knowledge about humankind as a whole, and of the particular patient and family concerned. It is impossible to know about every cultural system. However, it is desirable for a clinician to have some basic anthropological knowledge about how human beings vary in their habits, customs, beliefs, value systems, and illness behavior, in particular. They should know more about the cultural systems of the patients under care so that culture-relevant assessment and treatment can be delivered. Reading books and other literature is one way to obtain such cultural information. Consulting with medical anthropologists on general issues, or experts on a particular cultural system, is another approach. If such material or consultation is not easily available, the patient and his family or friends of the same ethnic-cultural background may be used as resources, even though careful judgment is needed in determining the accuracy and relevance.

Cultural Empathy

Factual information about a patient's culture alone is not sufficient to make a connection with the patient transculturally. There is another quality needed—namely, being able to feel and understand at an emotional level, from the patient's own cultural perspective. Otherwise, a gap in understanding will remain still, and the clinicians will be unable to participate in and understand the emotional experience of the patient. *Cultural empathy* refers to the ability to develop an empathic understanding at an emotional level so that a true connection can be made, which, in turn, often allows the most appropriate care to be rendered. This is particularly true for mental health care and conducting psychological counseling, but is also useful for healthcare in general.

Culturally Relevant Relations and Interactions

In a clinical setting, a healthcare practitioner seeks to establish a helpful, professional relationship with the patient, minimizing any complications or ill effects from that relationship. The age, gender, and personality of the patient, the hierarchical aspect of the relationship, the nature and severity of the medical problems, and the purpose of care are some of the elements to consider in adjusting this relationship. As an extension of this, there is a need to incorporate cultural attributes. The clinician should take into consideration the cultural background of the patient, the clinician's own cultural background, and cultural aspects of the setting in which the care takes place.

Culturally Appropriate Health Care Delivery

In addition to providing *medically* appropriate care of the patient, the healthcare provider needs to assess and consider whether the care delivered to the patient is *culturally* suitable or not. When performing an obstetric or a gynecologic examination for a patient from Micronesia, it would be culturally appropriate for the clinician to invite the patient's husband or female family member to be present during the examination. When proposing an amputation of an extremity for an Asian or Arabic patient, the surgeon needs to be aware of what it might mean to a patient whose culture emphasizes the integrity of the whole body for future life. To prescribe alcohol-containing liquid medicine, the clinician needs to know that this may not be welcome by some Muslim patients who avoid intake of alcohol due to their religious beliefs. Alternative medication should be considered to avoid the conflict with the patient's taboo. Ideally, the clinician should select clinically and culturally suitable methods of treatment to best serve the patient.

Cultural Guidance

If cultural factors are part of the patient's health problems, or interfere with medical treatment, culturally relevant advice for patients in dealing with their problems may be needed. Culturally determined norms, values, and goals may not always be able to be accommodated. They may need to be challenged and adjusted in order to treat problems or resolve conflicts. Culturally sanctioned coping mechanisms may need reinforcement, or, if ineffective, may need to be confronted. Alternatives to culturally defined solutions may need to be proposed. It takes not only clinical judgment but cultural insight to find relevant and optimal solutions.

Awareness of Healthcare Provider's Own Culture

It is vital to know that the performance of healthcare involves the interaction of two value systems—the patient's and the clinician's. The method of care, the direction of treatment, and the outcome of care that is aimed for may depend on the clinician's medical judgment, but in subtle or even explicit ways, may be influenced by the healthcare provider's own personality, individual viewpoints, and cultural bias. The healthcare provider does his or her best to constantly examine the degree to which medical decisions or recommendations reflect the provider's personal cultural values. For example, to encourage or discourage artificial abortion, to suggest surgical sterilization for the male, to advise having a hysterectomy—all potentially involve a clinician's personal view and cultural values regarding such medical procedures. It is the healthcare provider's responsibility to make sure that health care decisions are not biased by personal emotion and cultural values.

Medical Universality versus Cultural Relativism

Although it is important to provide healthcare that takes into account the patient's cultural background, this does not mean that the clinician needs to abandon appropriate medical care because of the patient's culture. If necessary, the clinician may work with and help the patient to accept a compromise between what is considered a universal truth medically and what the patient regards as specifically culturally appropriate. When a young child suffers from diarrhea and mild dehydration, manifesting signs of *fallen fontanelle* (*mollera caida*), it is unlikely to be helpful to the Mexican mother for the care provider to argue that it is wrong to worry about the sunken fontanelle, or to criticize the mother's folk method of treatment (placing salt on spots) as being silly and unnecessary. Rather, the clinician could concentrate on the assessment of the cause of diarrhea, correcting the dehydration, and educating the mother through the interpreter that the reason the child's fontanelle is fallen is due to the shortage of water from the excessive diarrhea, and that the primary goal of treatment is to stop the diarrhea and to provide sufficient water for the child. There does not have to be a contradiction between the mother's folk interpretation of the *illness* and the physician's concern with the *disease*. This can be seen as merely a different focus of attention and interpretation between the family and clinician—between universal medical knowledge and folk interpretation—that can be combined for the total care of the sick child.

Confronting Medically Dangerous Cultural Beliefs

Sometimes the patient's cultural belief not only does not match with the universal medical knowledge, but also interferes with necessary medical care. In such a situation, the healthcare provider should work with the patient to adjust the problematic cultural view and belief so that suitable healthcare can be provided. For example, if parents refuse life-saving blood transfusions for their child because of the religious beliefs of their community, it is the clinician's duty and responsibility to try and persuade the parents to bend their cultural belief to save the child's life. This can be done in stages. First, discussion with the parents should be tried because they may be ambivalent about their decision. Then, perhaps a family meeting can be scheduled or respected community leaders can be brought in to help the parents find a way to allow the needed treatment. If all else fails, legal action can be (and has been) used to save a life.

Another example would be parents that want their young daughter to have a female circumcision. It is appropriate for the physician to sensitively educate the parents that the world is changing, and it is important for women to have options in life and not merely be objects for men. In addition, female circumcision is painful with potential physical complications, and it risks psychological harm. Making good use of medical rationale to persuade the parents to rethink a maladaptive traditional ritual, and adapt to contemporary healthier values, is an honorable thing for the healthcare provider to do.

Cultural Considerations for Minorities

Associated with the ease of long-distance travel, migration is increasing, and societies around the world are becoming more multiethnic and polycultural. Healthcare providers are called upon to provide care for ethnic minorities, foreign migrants, international travelers, and indigenous peoples who are minorities.

As used here, the term *minority* refers to a group of people who, because of characteristics such as ethnicity, race, language, age, and physical handicap, are deprived of ordinary privileges enjoyed by the majority in the society. These can include access to healthcare services and quality of medical treatment. Minorities may encounter many obstacles to healthcare, including problems relating to and communicating with care providers. Minorities may have wide gaps with their healthcare providers in terms of cultural beliefs. Thus, providing culturally suitable care for minorities may require extra attention and effort.

Cultural Considerations for Every Patient and Family

In a broader sense, every individual has a unique background and different experiences to a greater or lesser degree. Thus, each patient can be seen as having a unique *culture* within a larger, more general culture. The principles of culturally competent care will, therefore, apply to all patients and families regardless of whether the patient is a minority or part of the majority, and whether he or she belongs to any particular ethnic or cultural group (Tseng & Streltzer 2004). Learning about culture and cultures—developing cultural sensitivity and understanding—will not only lead to culturally competent healthcare, but to competent healthcare in general.

References

Tseng WS (2003) Clinician's guide to cultural psychiatry. Academic Press, San Diego
Tseng WS, Streltzer J (2004) Cultural competence in clinical psychiatry. American Psychiatry Publishing, Washington D.C.

Index

About the Authors

Wen-Shing Tseng, M.D.

Wen-Shing Tseng, M.D., is a professor of psychiatry at the University of Hawaii School of Medicine. Born in Taiwan in 1935, he was trained in psychiatry at the National Taiwan University in Taipei, and later at the Massachusetts Mental Health Center of Harvard Medical School in Boston. He was a research fellow in culture and mental health at the East-West Center from 1970 to 1971 before being recruited as a faculty member of the University of Hawaii School of Medicine, where he became a professor in 1976 and served as training director for the psychiatric residency training program between 1975 and 1982.

As a consultant to the World Health Organization, as well as for teaching and research projects, he has traveled extensively to many countries in Asia and the Pacific, including China, Japan, Singapore, Malaysia, Fiji, and Micronesia. He served as chairman of the Transcultural Psychiatry Section of the World Psychiatric Association for two terms—from 1983 to 1993. In that capacity, he developed a wide network of colleagues around the world in the field of cultural psychiatry. He has coordinated numerous international conferences relating to the subject of culture and mental health in such places as Honolulu, Beijing, Tokyo, and Budapest, and recently cosponsored cultural psychiatry meetings in Kamakura, Japan and Stockholm, Sweden.

He has conducted numerous research projects, mainly relating to the cultural aspects of assessment of psychopathology, child development, family relations, epidemic mental disorders, culture-related specific psychiatric syndromes, folk healing, and psychotherapy. The studies have resulted in the publication of more than 80 articles in scientific journals and chapters in books.

He has authored, edited, or co-edited nearly twenty books in English and more than thirty books in Chinese—mostly on the subjects of culture and mental health, culture and psychotherapy, and cultural psychiatry. Among them, the *Handbook of Cultural Psychiatry* (Academic Press, 2001) has received the Creative Scholar Award from the Society for the Study of Psychiatry and Culture. Some of his books have been translated into Japanese and Italian.

He has held the position of guest professor of the Institute of Mental Health at Peking University since 1987. He has been a Distinguished Life Fellow of the

American Psychiatric Association since 2003. He has served as an Honorable Advisor of the Transcultural Psychiatry Section of the World Psychiatric Association since 1996. Presently, he is the President of the World Association of Cultural Psychiatry, which was founded in 2005. Because of his research, publications, and experience, he has gained a reputation as one of the foremost experts in cultural psychiatry—at both national and international levels.

Jon Streltzer, M.D

Jon Streltzer, M.D., is a professor of psychiatry at the University of Hawaii School of Medicine, where he was training director from 1982–1996. A graduate of Yale University (B.A., philosophy) and the University of Colorado School of Medicine, he did a medicine internship at Queen's Hospital, Honolulu, and his psychiatry residency at Yale University School of Medicine. A Distinguished Life Fellow of the American Psychiatric Association, he is certified by the American Board of Psychiatry and Neurology in general psychiatry, addiction psychiatry, and pain management. A consultation-liaison psychiatrist, he organized the 17th World Congress on Psychosomatic Medicine in Waikoloa, Hawaii in 2003. He is President-elect of the International College of Psychosomatic Medicine, and Treasurer of the World Association of Cultural Psychiatry. He has published four books and more than 65 journal articles and book chapters in the areas of psychosomatic medicine, pain, and cultural psychiatry.

Printed in the United States
110373LV00003B/247-255/A